Patient -vs- Doctor

MISDIAGNOSIS

Written By:

Garry L. Jones

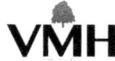

Manufactured in the United States of America

10 9 8 7 6 5 4 3 2 1

Hardback ISBN: 978-0-9979397-9-8

Paperback ISBN: 978-0-9984553-1-0

Cover Design Concept: Garry L. Jones

Cover Design: Vikki Hankins

Cover Image: Shutterstock

Editor: Terry Simms Wooten

Medical Terminology Advisor: Ronald Watson, PA-C

Author's Note:

This book is not intended as a substitute for the medical advice of
physicians. The reader should regularly consult a physician in
matters relating to his/her health and particularly with respect to
any symptoms that may require diagnosis or medical attention. The
names and characters have been changed to protect the privacy of
such individual's. The events documented in this public*ation are*
according to the author's memory. The publisher is not responsible
for websites (or their content) that are to owned by the publisher.

We are here by the mercy of God, my journey in life has given me a chance to open my eyes and walk a path that has given me a second chance at life. As you review the pages of this book you'll see the struggle for good health in my life, my frustrations, my disappointments, my hardships and my pain. As you review the pages you also see that we are all alike in many ways because my story is not unlike most people. Let me say that medicine is not an absolute science the esteemed specialists with advanced training and insight also make mistakes.

It is up to you to never accept normal as a diagnosis when you're having problems that you never had before and are unresolved. It is the responsibility of your physician to refer you to another physician who may know a little more about your problem if that physician is at an endpoint with your diagnosis. THE HIPPOCRATIC OATH states (if you can do no good, do no harm) the fact is laboratory tests do not diagnose a patient problem, they only confirm the diagnosis, the physician treats the patients not the test, there will always be false negative and false positives. It is the patient history and physical examination that make the diagnosis for the doctor. The fact that all these tests that I had to endure were necessary but misleading, misleading to indicate that nothing was wrong when I had cancer present in my prostate. I thank God every day (Lamentations 3: 22-23). It is of the Lord's mercies that we are not consumed fail not. They are new every morning great is thy faithfulness) only by God's mercy was I able to preserve and walked down the path of light that delivered me to my salvation (the Mayo Clinic in Jacksonville, Florida).

TABLE OF CONTENTS

CHAPTER 1

DID THE BURGER MAKE ME SICK?

The year was 1998, and it wasn't a good year for me. I had personal problems as well as health problems. I couldn't get rid of either one. The only thing good about that year was that I turned 35 years old. The saga begins.

Lieutenant John Coleman and I were Lieutenants at the Federal Correctional Institution/Federal Detention Center - Tallahassee in Tallahassee, Florida. We had gone to Rally's fast food joint. We both ordered a Big Buford and large fries; I think they had a special - buy one big Buford and get the second one free. When we got back to John's house, like always, John would put hot sauce on his fries, something I had never heard of. We both sat back and conversed about what was going on at the prison. It was getting kind of late, and I decided to go home. The next day for the next 13 years I would battle with an illness that had doctors baffled.

I awakened with a terrible headache; something I don't have often. When I urinated, it felt like someone had cut me with a razor blade. I was sweating profusely, and I felt chills all over my body. My lower back was hurting so bad that it was hard for me to stand up straight. I figured that I must have a virus or something because I never felt so bad. I can't recall how I got to the Tallahassee Community Hospital which is now called Capital Region. I think I may have taken myself because it was during the school year, and my children weren't around and neither was my ex-wife. By the time I arrived at the emergency room, I was in so much pain that I had to lie on the floor in a fetal position. After about an hour, I heard the name Garry Jones coming from a nurse telling me to come with her.

The nurse commenced to asking so many questions that it irritated me. I wanted to get out of this pain quick, fast, and in a hurry. The nurse took my temperature, and it was 104 degrees. She asked me to urinate in a cup, and I remembered asking what the purpose of that was. She stated, "With your symptoms Mr. Jones, it appears you may have Gonorrhea." "What in the hell do you mean that you think that I may have Gonorrhea," I shouted! "Calm down, Mr. Jones," she said, "we have to check and possibly rule that out," the nurse explained.

The only thing that I could think of was my ex-wife asking me why they took a test to see whether or not I had gonorrhea. In the back of my mind, I was thinking once she heard the word Gonorrhea, nothing and whatever I said next would register in her mind.

The doctor came in the room and said, "Mr. Jones, you have one of the worst urinary tract infections I've ever seen. Mr. Jones you also have blood in your urine." I said to the doctor, "I thought that only women got urinary tract infections." The doctor told me that men could get urinary tract infections as well but it's not as common as women. The doctor prescribed me some antibiotics and pain medication. After the pharmacist filled my prescription, he asked me a question. "Mr. Jones, do you have cancer?" I said, "No, why would you ask me a question like that?" He said, "The doctor put you on a large dose of OxyContin, and normally that's what cancer patients take when they are in pain. When I walked out of the pharmacy, I had an epiphany. I thought to myself that it must have been the Big Buford that I had eaten the night before because the doctor also said that I had a trace of e-coli.

I called John to see whether or not he had gotten sick, and he had not. "What's wrong Garry?" John asked. "John, I awaken this morning sick as hell. I went to the emergency room, and the doctor said that I had a trace of 100,000 E. coli and a urinary tract infection," I said. "I'm sorry to hear that Garry," he said, "and by the way, I'm on my way to get another Big Buford. Do you want one?" "Hell no, John," I replied.

The next week I went to my family physician. He examined me and noticed that I still had blood in my urine. He told me that if I have another urinary tract infection, he would have to send me to an urologist.

Two weeks later I developed another urinary tract infection. I awaken the next morning feeling fine. After I got off work, I went to the gym to get my work out on. When I left the gym, I could feel my lower back hurting, and my body began to feel raw all over. I couldn't tolerate anything touching my body. When I took a shower, I began to hurt. Even the water beating against my body felt as if I had fallen down on cement and gotten skinned all over. I thought to myself, I know I'm not having another urinary tract infection. A couple of hours later I went to the bathroom and started throwing up, and when I urinated it felt like my penis had been cut with a razor blade and alcohol was being poured over the tip of it. I began sweating profusely. I went to the emergency room, and like always they took my urine and tested me for Gonorrhea. I told them, again, that I was tired of them testing me for Gonorrhea. This time my ex-wife had taken me to the emergency room and she looked at me and asked, "Have you been messing around? Why would the doctors test you for Gonorrhea?" "I don't know," I told her. When the doctor came in the room, he told me that I had another bad urinary tract infection and confirmed my previous admission that the test for gonorrhea was negative. "No shit," I said! The doctor gave me another prescription for antibiotics and pain medication. I informed the doctor that I still had one or two antibiotic pills left as well as pain pills. He instructed me to complete the round of antibiotics and start a second round of antibiotics for a month. I asked the doctor, "Why do I have to continue to take these antibiotics, and why do I continue to get these urinary tract infections? What the hell is really going on?" The doctor looked at me without saying a word. I thought to myself does he even know what I have to go through when I get home. This woman is going to get all up in my face and start accusing me with some inaccurate information. My ex never failed when she was accusing me; it was just like clockwork. She would say, "Garry, who have you been messing with? You came home one night about 3:00 a.m. and said you had a flat tire and that's why you

13

were late. Then you said you were at a sports bar. Which one was it? I called all the sports bars, and the owner said that they closed at 2:00 a.m." "Look, dammit! When I did come home, I had a doughnut (temporary tire) on my car, and I had left the bar around 1:45 a.m. and that's when I got a flat tire," I said to her. My ex stated that I could have called, but it is not like we were on speaking terms. She would get pissed off when I drank alcohol at the house so I would go to sports bars to look at games and drink. My ex would say, "Yeah, you loved going to Hooters to look at the girls with those tight shorts on." Then I would say, "Look woman", when I do go to Hooters, I don't be looking at the girls with the tight shorts on. Those girls are a few years older than our daughter LaToya."

CHAPTER 2

THE END OF YEAR 1998

After taking my antibiotics I began to feel pretty good, but I was still afraid to eat at Rally's. I had begun to workout with vengeance. By now my family had left me, and I was all by myself. And once again, six months later, I became infected with another urinary tract infection. I went to bed feeling fine, then I awaken around 2:00 a.m. sick on the stomach and throwing up. And yes, just as before, when I urinated, I would burn so bad that tears streamed down my face. My body began to shut down, and I knew that something was seriously wrong with me. I went to the hospital again, and it was the same routine. The nurse would say, "Mr. Jones, we are going to test you for Gonorrhea. Could you provide us with a sample of your urine?" I gave the nurse what she asked for, and I told her that she was not going to find Gonorrhea; but she would find a urinary tract infection. I asked her to give me something for my pain. The doctor walked in and said that I had tested negative for Gonorrhea, but he had noticed that I had a

15

bad urinary tract infection. He told me to go home and drink plenty of Cranberry juice and water and take my antibiotics until completion. I said, "Doctor, I'm sick and tired of being sick. Do you know what is causing all of these urinary tract infections?" "No, Mr. Jones," he replied. I thought to myself that they don't know anything. That is why they call them all practicing physicians because they practice on people instead of curing them. I'm tired of being their guinea pig. I went home, got back in bed, and continued taking antibiotics every day for two months. I guess a burger wasn't making me sick.

CHAPTER 3

2000 IS GOING TO BE A GOOD YEAR

I can recall rumors going around about how the computers were going to mess up when the clock struck 12. Some people were saying the world was going to end, and it did for some people because a lot of people died in the year 2000. And just like the previous years, my urinary tract infections kept coming back. Finally my family physician recommended that I go to see an urologist. On January 3, 2000, I had an appointment to see Doctor Bird at the Southeastern Urological Center. I was at the office around 9:00 a.m. for a consultation. He asked permission to do a prostate exam, and I agreed but wasn't happy because I hated those finger waves. I have had more than my share, and I was only 35 years of age. Doctor Bird asked me if my testicles hurt when I got sick, and I told him no.

This was Doctor Bird's assessment of me:

Mr. Jones is a 35 year old black male referred by Dr. Waterford for evaluation of blood in his urine. Doctor Waterford noted Mr. Jones having blood in his urine on several occasions. Patient also has a history of greater than 100,000 E. coli urinary tract infections in January of 1999. The patient's genitourinary history is remarkable in that he denies excessive frequent urination and nocturia. He denies gross blood. He denies multiple recurrent urine infections.

After reading the report in which the doctor had documented that I had denied having frequent urine infections, I figured he must have gotten me mixed up with another patient. The reason I was referred to him was because of the blood and urine infection. Dr. Bird was arrogant and didn't like for anyone to ask him questions. He had, like many doctors have, a God Complex.

Dr. Bird would soon find out that I asked a lot of questions when it came to my body, and if you are reading this book, I would urge you to ask a lot of questions, too. Some doctors like to shrug you off when you ask questions as if you are challenging them.

Follow Up Visit

On January 14, 2000, I returned to Dr. Bird for a follow-up visit. I had come prepared because I knew what procedure he was going to perform. This procedure gave me hope because it was going to show what was going on with my kidneys and prostate. He performed a Cystoscopy and IVP. A Cystoscopy is a very uncomfortable procedure. I was awake for the cystoscopy. A cystoscopy, or cystourethroscopy, is an endoscopic procedure where a tube is inserted into the urethra through the opening at the end of the penis. It allows the doctor to visually examine the complete length of the urethra and the bladder for tumors, strictures, prostate enlargement, and other problems.

During the procedure, water is inserted through the cystoscope and into your bladder. Your healthcare provider will ask you a series of questions about how you feel while your bladder is filled. When the bladder is full of water, it stretches. This allows your physician to view the entire bladder wall.

If any tissue appears abnormal, a biopsy (tissue sample) can be taken through the cystoscope to be analyzed.

The entire procedure, including preparation, generally takes about 15 to 20 minutes. The examination portion of the procedure is generally less than 5 minutes in duration.

As I mentioned earlier an IVP was performed as well. An intravenous pyelogram (IVP) (Image) Dye Test is an X-ray test that provides pictures of the kidneys, the bladder, the ureters, and the uretha (urinary tract). An IVP can show the size, shape, and position of the urinary tract, and it can evaluate the collecting system inside the kidneys.

During IVP, a dye called Contrast Material is injected into a vein in your arm. A series of X-ray pictures is then taken at timed intervals.

IVP is commonly done to identify diseases of the urinary tract, kidney stones, tumors, or infection. It is also used to look for problems with the structure of the urinary tract that were present from birth (congenital).

Dr. Bird's assessment of the procedure is as follows:

After being injected with IV contrast there are no immediate complications. There is prompt filling and draining of both collecting systems. There are no renal contour abnormalities. Mr. Jones will have a follow-up visit on October 20, 2000.

CHAPTER 4

OH NO! NOT AGAIN

It was May 2000, and I was on my way to the Post Office on Adams Street in Tallahassee, Florida. I began to feel my lower back aching, and when I got back home I could feel the rawness of my entire body. I couldn't sit down because I was hurting all over. I began to feel a headache coming, and when I went to use the bathroom I dreaded it. I knew when I began to urinate that I was going to burn like hell. The doctor's office was closed, so I was forced to go to the emergency room. When I arrived at the emergency room, I knew how the routine was going to go. Mr. Jones we need to get a urine sample; are you allergic to anything; no I'm not. Then the nurse said, again, "Can I take your temperature please? You feel like you are burning up, and I can see you are in an excruciating amount of pain." "Have you had this problem before?" she asked. "Yes, about five times already," I replied. "We have to check to see whether or not you have a Sexual Transmitted Disease, and we need to do a culture," she continued. I said, "Ma'am I don't have an STD. What I have is a bad urinary tract infection." "Why do you think that, Mr. Jones?" the nurse asked again. "Ma'am, I come in here all the time for the same problem." "Do you have an urologist?" I asked. "Yes, we do, she responded." "When was the last time you saw him?" the nurse inquired. "I saw him two months ago," I told her.

After all the repeated questions by the nurse, she informed me that the doctor would be with me shortly. I asked if I could have something to drink, but the nurse told me not until the doctor determined what was going on. The doctor came in and said, "Hello Mr. Jones. You don't look so well." "Sir, I don't feel well either," I replied. "We got your results back," he began. "You have one of the worst urinary tract infections I've seen. We are going to start you on some Cipro and give you some pain medication. I want you to follow-up with your Urologist," he continued. "I want you to drink plenty of water and Cranberry juice because Cranberry juice is good for urinary tract infections." I left the emergency room pissed. One doctor had already told me that it was not common for a man to have so many urinary tract infections, but no one was trying to find out what the cause of these urinary tract infections. Nevertheless, I took the medication as prescribe, and for the next couple of days I felt better.

CHAPTER 5

5 URINARY TRACT INFECTIONS WITHIN 18 MONTHS

On October 20, 2000, I had another follow-up appointment with my urologist. Needless to say, I wasn't thrilled. I only wanted to know what was going on with me. I know my sickness was not in my head because if that was the case I wouldn't have a high temperature. I kept asking myself why it burned every time I urinated, why my body ached all over, and why the hell did my results come back indicating that I had a urinary tract infection. When the nurse called me in the back to meet with the doctor, I didn't have a smile on my face. I informed the doctor that I had gotten sick again over the weekend

This was his assessment:

Gary returned to the office for follow-up today. He recently had another urinary tract infection which sounds like it may have been a prostatatits. He was treated at Tallahassee Memorial Hospital. There are no records and apparently he did not have a

culture obtained. He took Cipro for a few days but that made him feel bad and so he has just completed a course of Septra for a month. He feels markedly better.

IMPRESSION/PLAN: Probable prostatatitis. If patient develops recurrent symptoms I have asked him to come to our office so that I can evaluate him personally. Urinalysis today is normal. Previous IVP and cystoscopy have been normal.

I didn't know who was transcribing Doctor Bird's notes, but they couldn't spell worth a shit! I wished I had these notes earlier. I would have caught all the errors then I would have evaluated him and concluded that he wasn't the doctor for me. Doctors don't expect patients to ask for their medical records. I think a patient should always ask for their medical records to see what the doctor is putting in them. You will be amazed.

CHAPTER 6

PATIENT -VS- DOCTOR

It was November 27, 2000, and I had an appointment with Dr. Bird. I was determined to find out what was wrong with me, or I was going to ask for a second opinion. This particular day was where everything got heated between me and the doctor. I asked the doctor what was the root cause of my problem, and why was I continuing to get urinary tract infections. "Are you being promiscuous?" the doctor asked. "What the hell you just ask me?" I responded. "Are you being promiscuous?" the doctor repeated. "No, I'm not, and even if I were, don't you know I would have stopped had I known that was the root of my problem," I said. "Why in the hell would you ask me a question like that? Is it because you don't know what the hell is wrong with me so you are going to put the blame back on me?" I continued. Then Doctor Bird said, "You are in pretty good shape, and you are young. You aren't supposed to be having these urinary tract infections. The problems you are having are the problems I see in 60 and 70 year old patients," he stated. My response was, "Well, the fact of the matter is I'm still getting sick. I'm tired of taking your antibiotics and continue to get sick. I need to find out what is causing me to get sick. Now you are telling me you don't need to look any further. So, I'm telling you I'm going to get a second opinion, Dr. Bird!!!!"

Doctor Bird's Assessment:

Gary is a 36 year old black male whom I have been following for the past year. He has a history of recurrent UTI"'s, and has had what I believe is recurrent prostatitis . The patient recently had recurrence of some symptoms of a UTI with burning on urination and suprapubic discomfort. He was seen in the emergency room this past Friday. A urine culture, however, was not obtained. He was placed on Tequin, but has been having some sensitivity to this. In general, he is sensitive to Cipro and Fluorquinolones.

He then improved after a recent course of Septra X 30 days.

PHYSICAL EXAMINATION: A smooth abdomen which is soft. There is tenderness of the prostate, which is consistent with prostatitis.

The patient has had a normal IVP and cystoscopy within the last few months.

IMPRESSION: Recurrent prostatitis, possibly inadequately with Septra. The patient has been unable to tolerate fluoroquinolones, which are the No. 1 class of drugs to treat prostatitis.

PLAN: I have discussed the options with the patient. He is obviously frustrated, and I told him that I do not feel further studies are indicated at this time. We are going to try giving him Rocephin 500 mg IM QD X 7 days and then a full month of Trimethoprim. I'll see him back in 6 weeks for follow-up.

CHAPTER 7

SECOND OPINION

On December 08, 2000, I went to see Dr. James Cameo. He was a brother who stood over 6'2" tall with large hands. "I was reading your record, and you wanted to see me because you are not satisfied with Dr. Bird's assessment," he began. "You are right, Doctor Cameo. I'm not satisfied with Dr. Bird. Dr. Cameo, I want to know what is going on with my body," I responded. "I understand young man," he said. Then he told me to get undressed and bend over. Feeling a sense of violation coming on I said, "Dr. Cameo, I'm feeling alright today. So why do I have to keep getting the finger wave? I am tired of the doctors going up in me. It's been a year, and I have already had my prostate check at least six times. I'm beginning to think I'm not a man anymore." Dr. Cameo started laughing and said, "Everything is going to be alright." Dr. Cameo commenced to put his finger up my rectum, and I screamed, "Man this hurts!" Afterwards, Dr. Cameo and I had a long discussion of what might be going on with my prostate. I left his office feeling a little better, thinking maybe there was light at the end of the tunnel. However, after reading his notes, I realized that he was no different from Dr. Bird. All doctors stick together; I wonder do they take an oath not to go against one another.

Dr. Cameo's notes:

Mr. Jones comes in for a second opinion. He is a pleasant gentleman who has a history of having reoccurring and chronic urinary tract infections with prostatitis. He apparently had a documented E.coli infection. He has been treated with Trimethoprim and has been treated with IM Rocephin. He continues to have intermittent pain in the perineum, pain radiating to the low back, start/stop dribbling, and decreased force and caliber of the urinary stream. The patient says that he is no better. The patient has had work ups by Dr. Bird inclusive of IVP and cystoscopy which were basically normal. The patient was adamant today as to what was going on. He denies any fever or chills.

PHYSICAL EXAM: Alert and oriented.

Head/Neck: Normocephalic and atraumatic. Sclera and conjunctive are clear. Extraocular movements are full.

CHEST: Clear to auscultation. No rales or crackles.

CARDIAC: Normal S1 and S2 without appreciable murmur.

ANDOMEN: Soft, nontender. No palpable masses. No organomegaly. No inguinal adenopathy .

GENITOURINARY: Normal phallus. There are no meatal lesions.

No evidence of any scarring. Testes descended bilaterally without masses or tenderness. Cord structures are normal.

RECTAL: Normal spincter tone. Prostate is very, very, tender to palpation.

UA: pH 5, 0-5 WBC, 1 plus blood.

IMPRESSION: Acute prostatitis.

PLAN: I spent a long time discussing with the patient the fact that he may have reoccurring and chronic episodes of prostatitis and that he should expect to have this problem. Will treat him with Doxycycline and see him back in three months.

CHAPTER 8

BACK TO SQUARE ONE

On March 19, 2001, I had another infection, and I had to return to Dr. Bird as a walk-in because I got sick during business hours and didn't want to go to the emergency room. This was what Dr. Bird had to say:

Gary returns to the office as a walk-in today. He is a patient I have seen several times for recurrent episodes of prostatitis. He has recently seen Dr. Cameo for a second opinion. Dr. Cameo essentially had nothing new to add to my initial evaluation. The patient presents today with lower abdominal discomfort, burning on urination and dysuria. When he has an episode of prostatitis it is usually quite full blown and he is very symptomatic.

REVIEW OF SYSTEM: A per initial intake form of 01/03/2000 in the chart (See form) In addition to this he complains of burning dysuria. He denies hematuria. He reports frequent urination and pain in his perineal region. He denies any flank pain. He denies fever, chills, nausea and vomiting.

PHYSICAL EXAM: Reveals some tenderness in the suprapubic region. I did not perform a rectal exam for fear of causing aggravation of his symptoms and potentially precipitating some sepis.

UA: Nitrite positive urine, 20-40 white cells, 3 plus bacteria and occasional red cell.

IMPRESSION: Acute/chronic prostatitis.

PLAN: Gentamicin 80mg IM, Toradol 60mg, Cipro 500 mg BID for two months. Consider prostate ultrasound on patient's return.

Dr. Bird never performed the prostate ultrasound on patient's return.

CHAPTER 9

NEVER-ENDING CYCLE

I tried my best to keep myself in shape mentally, physically, and spiritually. I kept hope alive, but I was beginning to wear down. My resolve was weakening, and every day I told myself that I can't take but so much more of this. I was doing my part, but was my doctor doing his part. Was he doing everything possible to cure me? Was he consulting with other doctors to find out what they would do if given my medical information, or did he have too much pride to even ask? Dr. Bird kept telling me that I didn't have cancer, but I wondered if he ordered all the tests to rule cancer out. One day I was in his office and he said to me, "I could always rotor rutor you." I asked, "What does that mean?" He said, "We can take your prostate out." I responded, "Why would I have my prostate taken out when you can't find the root of the problem? Why remove an organ when you don't have to?" I told him that I would never agree to that. I compared his recommendation to a woman having pain then a doctor, not knowing what was wrong, takes her uterus out because she was having pain. When a woman's uterus or man's prostate have been removed, you have now prevented them from having any more children. I can only imagine how many doctors have removed organs from a human being because they didn't know what was going on, and after they removed the organ, the patient was still having the same problem. Not saying I wanted anymore children but that choice should be mine, not the doctors. Dr. Bird wanted to play Russian roulette with me, but I refused to play his game.

On May 24, 2001 I had another appointment with Dr. Bird, and these were his findings:

Gary returns to the office today for follow-up. He's had a recent recurrence of prostatitis. I gave him two months of antibiotics the last time I saw him, and he was only able to get through one month before getting sick. He has recently restarted on Cipro and is already feeling better in regards to his symptoms of prosatitis .

A recent PSA was 1.9 on April 22, 2001 figuring against possibility of prostate cancer causing his symptoms. Previous upper tract studies and cystoscopy have been normal

UA: Normal

We've decided to go ahead and have him complete his course of Cipro for this month. Then I'm going to put him on a suppressive antibiotic, Trimethoprim 100mg PO QD, and see him back in about three months for a follow-up.

It should be noted Dr. Bird didn't discuss with me my PSA (Prostate Specific Antigen) results. He always said it was within normal range. I knew that the PSA fluctuated and could be up one day and two days later it would be back within normal range. Even when my PSA was high, the doctor said it was normal. Why was he lying? Was it to keep me coming back to milk the insurance company? I didn't care about insurance companies because they rip patients off all the time. So if Dr. Bird would have charged the insurance company one million dollars for treating me, I wouldn't have given a damn because all I wanted was to be treated right and not lied to.

I encourage anyone who is reading this book to always request your medical records and see if the medical records match up with what the doctor told you in his office. And if the records don't match up, ask the doctor why would he tell you one thing and your medical records told you another thing.

CHAPTER 10

THE SAGA CONTINUES BETWEEN PATIENT AND DOCTOR

I was at the point where I was sick and tired of seeing Dr. Bird, with his God Complex. Whatever he said was the gospel; to hell with the patient. He didn't want to admit that he didn't know what was going on with my prostate, and he wanted me to continue to take antibiotics for the rest of my life. He stated that I had the flare-ups because I stopped taking the medication; hell, when I was taking medication, I still had the flare-ups. I understood that I had what he called prostatitis, but I didn't agree with his assessment when he stated that some patients get prostatitis, and there is nothing that doctors can do about it so the patients have to stay on antibiotics. The doctor failed to realize that once your body gets immune to certain antibiotics, they don't have the same effect anymore, and therefore, it is useless to continue to take them. I'm a firm believer that antibiotics cause other illnesses if taken a long time.

On May 01, 2002 I had another follow-up with Doctor Bird and his assessment was:

Gary returns to the office today for follow-up. He has had a recent flare prostatitis. He was started on Levaquin by Dr. Waterford's office. The patient is feeling better. He was having a fever up to 102 and now it is back down to about 100 degrees and he symptomatically is improved. When I saw him back in May of last year, he was having repeated flares, but had done better after completing a course of antibiotic and going on suppressive antibiotics with Trimethoprim q. h. s. The patient actually has not had any trouble for the last year until recently, and so is doing markedly better. He stopped his suppressive antibiotics and I suspect this the reason why he has had another flare up.

May 31, 2002, Gary returned to the office for follow-up. His symptoms of prostatitis. He also complains of ankle pain and leg pain he has been having for six months. His chief complaint today would be prostatitis. Gary wonders if Levaquin side effects causes leg and ankle pain.

June 06, 2002 Gary PSA is 0.74 normal range.

August 30, 2002 Gary returns to the office today for follow-up. He has a history of prostatitis and that is why he is here today. He also had a recent PSA performed and is here to follow-up for the results. His most recent PSA is 0.74.

CHAPTER 11

2.35 PROSTATE SPECIFIC ANTIGEN IS NOT THE NORM FOR ME

It had been three years since my first encounter with Dr. Bird, and it appeared that we were not getting anywhere. I didn't know what was going on in my body, and he didn't know what was going on either. Some doctors would recommend their patients to another doctor if they couldn't solve the problems. Doctors should care about the patients, and if they can't help them, then maybe someone else can.

It's April 10, 2003 at 11:30 a.m., and I was at Doctors Bird's office for another follow-up:

Gary returns for follow-up. He has had some recurrent symptoms of prostatitis and has been on Levaquin for two weeks with improvement in his symptomatology. He is back today just for a routine follow-up. He wonders why he keeps getting prostatitis. I have told him some individuals simply get prostatitis. His PSA's have been normal. His rectal exams have been normal other than some tenderness. His cystoscopy was normal. I don't see any anatomic basis for these recurrent infections. Some patient does simply get this. I have told him that as I have recommended previously, we could put him on a suppressive antibiotic nightly to keep these infections from recurring. In the past he has not wanted to do that. He actually has done well since August and just recently got this infection and so almost eight months have elapsed since his last bout with prostatitis. I have again discussed risk factors of getting prostatitis and I don't see that he falls into any of those categories particularly.

The day prior, April 09, 2003, at 11:15 a.m. blood was drawn from my arm for the purpose of getting a PSA. (Prostate Specific Antigen) The test came back 2.35. This was not in the normal range for me.

Dr. Bird never discussed my PSA results with me. The only reason I know about the PSA is because I'm reading his notes. These are Dr. Bird notes- not mine.

June 15, 2003, would be my last appointment with Doctor Bird. September 01, 2003, I moved to Atlanta, Georgia.

CHAPTER 12

SICK IN ATLANTA

I moved to Atlanta, and my physical problems moved as well. After living in Atlanta for six months, I became very ill one night. I began to sweat profusely, and my head was pounding. When I went to the restroom and began to urinate, I almost dropped to my knees because of the severe pain and burning sensation. It wasn't a secret; I knew that I had another urinary tract infection. I had given up on going to the doctor or the emergency room. I reached for my medical bag, grabbed my antibiotics and pain killers, and treated myself for 15 more days.

Two weeks had passed, and I awaken feeling great. I decided to go for my morning stroll, and in the middle of my stroll I became very ill in a matter of seconds. My back and lower back began to hurt, but I attributed the problem to having too much weight around my midsection. I walked for another half of a mile but my head continued to pound, and my body began to feel raw all over. I said out loud, "I can't

45

believe that I have another urinary tract infection." "I'm sick of this!" "Why in the hell do I continue to have these urinary tract infections?" "I'm too young to be this sick, especially since I take care of myself," I yelled!

I was able to make it back home. When I arrived I went on the internet to find me an urologist in Atlanta. I found one in midtown Atlanta and made an appointment. A few days later I was in his office writing down all of my medical issues. The doctor stated, "Mr. Jones, given your history of recurring urinary tract infections and what you are telling me, it appears all the right test have been conducted." "Do you think your infection has gone away considering you last had it a couple of days ago?" he asked. "No, Doc. I'm sure I'm still sick," I replied. The doctor went out of the room, and five minutes later a beautiful African American nurse came in the office and handed me a cup. I knew what the cup was for.

She continued to smile. I asked myself why in the hell was she smiling. I thought that this sister must have a crush on me, but then again she didn't know who I was, and I'm sure the doctor had shared with her what was going on with me. She said, "Mr. Jones, we need a sample." I said, "Where is the restroom?" She pointed over in the corner. When I went to the room to give a urine sample, there was no toilet. I asked, "Ma'am, where is the toilet?" She responded, "There is no toilet in that room." "How am I'm going to give my urine sample?" I asked. "Mr. Jones, did the doctor tell you what kind of sample he wanted?" she asked. I said, "No, he didn't. He just walked out of the room then you came in." The nurse finally figured out that I had no clue as to what the hell was going on.

"Mr. Jones, we need a semen sample," she said. "You need a what," I replied. "We need to get some semen from you," she repeated. I said, "How do you expect to get some semen from me? What kind of mess is this? Is the doctor a freak?" I wasn't smiling anymore. I became down right angry. She said, "Mr. Jones, we need that semen." However, the way she said it made me think that she was a freak. I asked, "How are you going to get some semen from me?" She pointed to the room again and walked over there with me. She said, "This room has plenty of playboy magazines." I asked, "Magazines for what? Oh. Are you saying you want me to masturbate in this cup?" She then started laughing instead of smiling. She responded, "That is usually the way we get your semen. Yes, you masturbate in the cup, and we take the sample and send it to the lab." "Ma 'am, you must be out of your damn mind," I said angrily. "So, I guess you are going to look?"

47

I asked. She started laughing again. I said, "The shit ain't funny, and I'm not doing it."

The nurse left the room, and the doctor came back in and said, "Mr. Jones, if you don't feel comfortable masturbating in the office, take the cup home, and after you have finished take the semen to a Lab Corp. Here is the paperwork to give to the personnel," he told me. I walked out of the office feeling like I had just been violated, mentally.

CHAPTER 13

LABCORP VISIT

One Saturday morning I called a Labcorp in Riverdale, Georgia to see whether or not they opened on the weekend. The receptionist said they were open but closed at 12:00 noon. I got in my car and drove to Lapcorp with my semen in a cup sealed in a plastic bag. I was so embarrassed. I arrived at the office and went to the receptionist desk and said, "I'm Mr. Jones." She said, "Yes, I remember I talked with you about 35 minutes ago, Mr. Jones." "What do you have for me?" she asked. I whispered in her ear, "I have some semen for you." She started smiling and said, "Mr. Jones, you don't have to feel embarrassed. We get those samples every day. As a matter of fact, you are the third person to drop some off." "Do you have the paperwork from the doctor?" she asked, and I said, "Yes I do." She said, "It will take about two to three days to test, then we will send the results to the doctor." The receptionist said in a facetious tone, "You have a nice day Mr. Jones, and hopefully everything will turn out alright."

While on my way home, I had a lot of thoughts that were going in and out of my mind. I thought, maybe the doctor can find out what was going on. Maybe he didn't need a urine sample. I figured when the test results came back, he would be able to really tell me what was wrong.

Tuesday morning I received a called from my doctor's office. The nurse told me that my tests had come back, and the doctor wanted to know if he could see me in a couple of days. I asked, "How about today?" The nurse replied, "Let me put you through to the receptionist to see whether or not the doctor can see you today." I waited on the line, and the nurse returned to the phone and said, "Mr. Jones, the doctor can see you tomorrow morning at 9:30 a.m." I said, "Great. I will be there."

The next day I arrived at the doctor's office not knowing what to expect. I went to the desk and said, "I'm Garry Jones. I'm here to see Dr. Wilson." "Have a seat, Mr. Jones. The doctor will be with you in a minute," the receptionist replied. Ten minutes later the same African American nurse that I had met before entered the room and said, "Dr. Wilson will see you now, Mr. Jones." The nurse and I engaged in small talked before she left the room. Dr. Wilson came in and asked, "How do you feel Mr. Jones?" "I'm fine. What about yourself, Dr. Wilson?" I responded. "I'm doing ok, Mr. Jones," he replied.

Dr. Wilson said, "Mr. Jones, I have your test results, and I must say, I've never seen a urinary tract infection this bad before." I said, "I think I have heard these words from another doctor in Florida, but just your words are not solving my problem." "I need to know what is going on," I said. "Mr. Jones, we are going to prescribe you another kind of antibiotic. If it doesn't make the infection go away, I want you to make an appointment to see me again," the doctor said. I walked out of the doctor's office, as usual, pissed; I knew I wasn't coming back, even if I was on my death bed.

CHAPTER 14

JOHN HOPKINS HOSPITAL

Even though I walked out of the doctor's office feeling dejected, I knew something foreign in my body was causing me to continue to get sick. I knew there were a lot of good hospitals in the United States, but John Hopkins was known to be one of the best. I could have gone back home to North Carolina and made an appointment either at Duke University Hospital or the University of North Carolina, but I needed to take a trip to Washington, D.C. to take care of some advocacy work, and this trip would give me an opportunity to visit my family in the DMV (D.C., Maryland, and Virginia) area.

I called one of my buddies who stayed in the DMV area, and informed him that I was going to make an appointment for medical reasons at John Hopkins University Hospital. "When is the appointment, Jones?" he asked. "Man, didn't I just tell you I was getting ready to make the appointment," I replied. "Sometimes I feel as though all you smart guys don't have any common sense," I said. He responded, "The reason I was asking, Jones, is because I want you to come and speak at Montgomery College." "Dr. Walter Fauntroy, former U.S. House of Representative and Civil Rights activist from Washington, D.C., will be the guest speaker, and I want you to be on the panel." He continued, "You can explain to the kids about mandatory minimum sentencing and maybe you can rub elbows with the congressman. Jones you know you love politics." "Man, let me get back with you on that," I said.

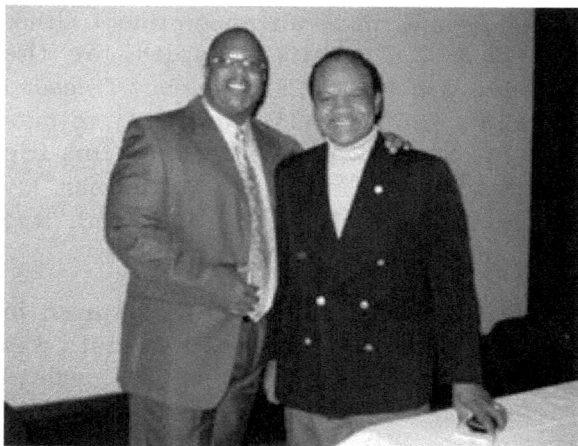

Garry Jones with Dr. Walter Fauntroy
(Former U.S. House of Representatives)

Mock Civil Rights Summit Program

We want to thank ALL students, faculty,
and guests for making the
College Institute Program's
2005 Mock Civil Rights Summit
a BIG SUCCESS!

2005 Summit
Organizers
Garrett Austen
Jeff Dimon
Daniel Gopenko
Josh Hackenberg
Neema Nassiri
Peter Sklaver
Alexander Tebeleff

Chairman
Professor M. V. Parker

Chairman Assistants
Emily Baden
Deborah Moldover
Lauren Rossnan

55

After talking with my buddy, I called John Hopkins University to make an appointment with the Urology and Gastroenterology doctors. I got damn lucky!!! They said they could see me in two weeks, and that was around the time my buddy wanted me to speak. I called my buddy back and said, "I have an appointment at John Hopkins around the time you wanted me to speak." "Jones, whether you could have gotten the appointment or not I had already put you on the program," he said. He told me, "Hey Jones, you have only five minutes to speak." I replied, "Man I can't give a damn speech on a sensitive subject like the draconian mandatory minimum sentencing drug laws in five minutes." "Well, Jones. You can't use more time than the guest speaker," he said. "Look, I said. "I understand where you are coming from, and I appreciate you inviting me to speak but at least give me ten minutes." "Bye Jones. We will talk about that when you get here," he replied.

I booked my flight to B.W.I. (Baltimore, Washington International Airport), and two weeks later I was in Baltimore, Maryland. My buddy picked me up from the airport, and we went back to his place to discuss the plans for me to speak at Montgomery College. The next day we arrived on campus, and there were more people from the outside than I expected. Needless to say, I was excited to meet Congressman Fauntroy. The program was awesome, and I kept my speech to seven minutes. I must say that wasn't the best speech I had ever given, but the children liked it. One of the parents came up to me afterwards and told me that I delivered some informative information.

My buddy and I arrived at John Hopkins University Hospital for my appointments. I first met with the gastroenterologist. He was a foreigner. I can't recall what country he was from but he appeared to be very nice. The doctor began, "Mr. Jones, I was reading your medical records, and it appears you have been having problems with your intestine, and this has caused discomfort." "You are absolutely right," I replied. He asked, "Mr. Jones, what are your major concerns?" I responded, "Well, doctor, I have noticed whenever I go to the restroom, I'm seeing more blood after I wipe myself. Also, sometimes my stomach hurts so bad it causes me to drop to my knees because of the severity of the pain." The doctor instructed me to take off my clothes and put on my gown. He informed me that he would be back with me later. When the doctor returned to my room to examine me, he noticed the blood that I had spoken of earlier. He asked me if I had a family history of diverticulitis, and I told him that I did. He told me that I was too young to be having these problems, and eventually I would have major problems with my colon. He then said, "Y'all don't have the proper diet." "What the hell you mean by y'all?" I angrily asked. The doctor immediately corrected himself and said Americans.

He said, "Americans eat a lot of fried, greasy spicy food with a lot of salt, and that is not good for your colon." "Mr. Jones, with the proper diet, I can help you get back on track." he stated. He continued, "I don't want you to eat any corn or spicy foods, and I want you to drink plenty of water. I want you to eat as much fiber as you can." He asked, "Mr. Jones, have you ever heard of Metamucil?" "Yes, I have doc," I responded. He said, "Take some every night." "How long do you want me to take the Metamucil?" I asked. The doctor replied, "Mr. Jones, you can take Metamucil for the rest of your life." "But doctor, I don't want to be on medication all of my life," I said. The doctor explained to me that Metamucil was not considered as medication, but rather it was a fiber. He continued, "Mr. Jones, I also want you to take two hot baths a day. This will help with the colon." The doctor assured me that if I followed his prescribed plan, he couldn't guarantee that I wouldn't have any more problems with my colon, but this plan would help reduce the problems with my colon especially as I get older.

Later on in the afternoon I had an appointment with the Urologist. I submitted all the prior paperwork from the other Urologist that I had seen in the past. The nurse entered and said, "Mr. Jones, the doctor will see you now." The first thing the doctor asked was, "Mr. Jones, what brings you here?" My response was, "If I'm not mistaken doctor, all of my medical paperwork was faxed to you, and I also have copies with me." I thought to myself that this doctor had not read anything, and if I wouldn't have informed him that I resided in Atlanta, he would have thought that I was a local patient. He asked to see my medical paperwork so that he could review it.

After reading some of my medical paperwork, the doctor informed me that he had to leave to attend a meeting, and he stated that from what he reviewed in my paperwork, he agreed with the rest of my doctors and their recommendation that I should continue to take antibiotics whenever I become infected with a urinary infection. He then proceeded to ask me, "Don't they have good doctors in Atlanta?" I said, "Sure, but I wanted to get a third and fourth opinion. I have been sick for a long time."

After leaving the doctor's office I was pissed, yet again. I wondered how the world renowned John Hopkins Hospital could employ such arrogant doctors like the one I had just seen. Needless to say, I got the name of his supervisor and wrote a detailed letter explaining my dissatisfaction with his doctor. A week after I arrived back in Atlanta, I received a call from the doctor's supervisor asking me how we could resolve the problems I had experienced at John Hopkins. I explain to him that in my opinion, before a doctor sees a new patient, and he has previously requested the new patient's medical records to be sent to him, he should at least read the records prior to the patient coming into his office. I'm sure there are great doctors at John Hopkins University, but unfortunately I was seen by a jackass. In preparation to writing this book, I requested my medical records from John Hopkins University. I will send a copy of my book to the urologist doctor that examined me.

Everyone should have a copy of their medical records just in case, when filing a complaint with about a doctor, the medical records come up missing.

CHAPTER 15

GREAT ADVICE

On September 15, 2007, I drove to Charlotte, North Carolina to meet up with my brother in order to catch a ride to New York. My nephew Terry Jones Jr. was a freshman at Elizabeth City State University, and my first cousin Carlos Hardy was playing for my alma mater at North Carolina Central University. They were playing in the 37th Annual Whitney Young Football Classic at Giants Stadium. My brother and I were excited.

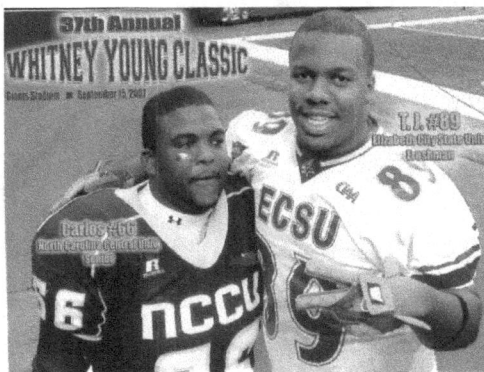

Carlos Hardy (Cousin) and Terry "T.J. Jones," Jr. (Nephew)

We received a call from another first cousin of ours, Comedian Garrick Dixon. Garrick was performing at THE IMPROV in Washington, D.C. He was doing big things traveling all over the world, performing live at the Apollo and playing in a part on the television series "Heroes". He also performed on the Jimmy Kimmel show, played in the television series show "All of Us", played a part in the R&B soul singer's Macy Grace video and was in Rap Superstar Little Wayne's video biggest hit song "How to Love." Garrick also performed on the Tony Rock Project;" the Superman commercial sponsored by Hardees/Carl's Jr. franchise; the Joan and Mellissa Rivers Show and was in many more roles. Our family was proud of him.

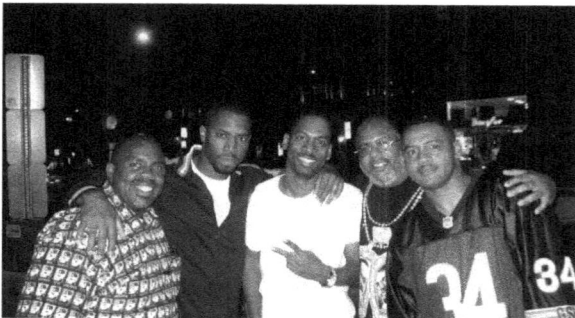

Terry Jones, Garrick Dixon, Tony Rock, Me, Sheldon (Shellcat)

The DMV area was a second home for us. My brother and I used to reside in

Maryland. I phoned Shellcat, a childhood friend of ours who also resided in the DMV area, to let him know that we should be hitting the area around 7:00 p.m.

I was excited about seeing Garrick because I hadn't seen him since his mother passed a year prior. Garrick was also from the DMV area but currently resided in California. We arrived in Washington, D.C. later than we had anticipated, and we called Shellcat to meet us on Connecticut Avenue where the IMPROV was located. When we got there the lines were long, but we didn't have to worry because we all were special guests of Garrick. When I saw Garrick, I gave him a great big hug; we were both still hurting from the loss of his mother and the loss of my aunt. We had the pleasure of meeting Tony Rock, the brother of Chris Rock. He and Garrick were the best of friends, and Garrick was opening for him. Garrick told us not to sit up front because the comedians would pounce on the audience that was sitting close to the stage.

The show started and it was hilarious. We all had a great time. After the show my brother Pete and I went over to our mother's place in Oxen Hill, Maryland. We were tired and needed to get some sleep. We woke up the next morning and headed over to D.C. to pick up Shellcat then headed to New York to see the game. Needless to say, my nephew and my cousin put on a show at the game; however, someone had to lose, and it was Elizabeth City State University. After the game we met with our relatives and told them how proud we were to see them play. Then we headed back to Washington, D.C.

The next day I called one of my classmates that stayed in the area. As a matter of fact, we used to date in high school but split up in 1979 and remained good friends until this very day. I went over to her house to see her, and she had prepared a meal. We laughed and talked, and I was telling her about my problems with my prostate. I told her that I had gone to so many doctors, but they couldn't find out what was wrong with me. She said, "Garry, why don't you go to the Mayo Clinic? You frequent Tallahassee a lot." I said, "The Mayo clinic is in Rochester, Minnesota." She stated, "They also have one in Jacksonville, Florida and Phoenix, Arizona." While working in the Bureau of Prisons, I used to transport inmates to Rochester but didn't have a clue there was a Mayo Clinic in Florida. After leaving my classmate's place, my brother and I went back to Charlotte, N.C. I picked up my car and drove back to Atlanta, Georgia. The advice I received from my classmate probably saved my life.

CHAPTER 16

MEDICARE

Shortly after winning my social security case on April 06, 2010, I was mentally exhausted. I had been fighting this case for seven years. It wouldn't have taken my case as long of a time to win if I had conformed to what the Government wanted me to do. I was being advised by my doctors to go out and participate in activities that I enjoyed but not to overdo it. My attorney was telling me otherwise which was to wait until my case went before court before I commenced to doing volunteer work. On the one hand, if I would have listened to what my attorney wanted me to do, I would have been in the insane asylum. So I took my doctors' advice and created my organization called Advocate4justice. I realized that the human body was built to do some form of activities whether it's physical exercising or whether it's exercising the brain. Just because a person may be declared disable, doesn't mean he/she is supposed to sit around and just collect a check each month. A person is to do some type of work, if not their body is going to waste away.

August 01, 2010, I received my Medicare card as well as the Medicare pamphlet. I read something in the pamphlet that caught my attention. It stated as long as you are on Medicare you are only entitled to one physical. Surely, this had to be a mistake. I figured that they must have meant one physical per calendar year. I called the Medicare office and asked one of the representatives was it true what I had read about being entitled to one physical as long as I'm on the medical program. The representative said, "Mr. Jones, what you read was correct. Medicare pays for only one physical as long as you are under Medicare." You would think that all medical programs would want any patient to have a physical every year for preventative measure, but I forgot this was a government program, and even Medicare had a lot of red tape. I was used to the bureaucracy. I had won one battle with the government only to be introduced to another one. This had been my life story, but I was well equipped to handle battles. God prepared me a long time ago how to fight my battles. Most of the time I didn't listen, but after God kept putting that belt to my behind, eventually I would recognized that God's way is the proper way, and if I just waited on that man, he would come through for me. I had to learn that the hard way.

Now my prayer goes a little something like this:

"God I come to you in the name of Jesus and the blood. I asked that you forgive me for my sins, iniquity, and transgressions. God I asked that your will be done in my life instead of my will. God, although I want my will to be done, I realized your will is the best way. God, I would love to have plenty of money in the bank and have a beautiful house to stay in and drive a nice car. But if this is not what you want for me, please provide me with the means to pay for what I have and to learn to appreciate all that you have given me. I pray this in your son's name Jesus, amen."

After getting off the phone with the Medicare agent, I decided that if I'm going to be allowed to have only one physical, then I would go to the best medical facility in the world to have my physical, and that was the Mayo Clinic located in Jacksonville, Florida. The one located in Jacksonville Florida was close to where I reside in Atlanta; the trip was only 5 hours away.

CHAPTER 17

ARRIVING AT THE WORLD RENOWNED
MAYO CLINIC

I called the Mayo Clinic to make an appointment for a physical. When the receptionist answered my call she asked, "What Physician referred you to the Mayo Clinic?" I said, "I referred myself. Is this going to be a problem?" "No, Mr. Jones, but we are backed up for a year," she replied. My heart dropped. The receptionist said, "If you would like, I can go ahead and take all your insurance information and put you on the waiting list. And if we have someone to cancel an appointment, we will give you a call. However, in the meantime, if there is something urgent you may need, I advise you to consult your medical personnel in Atlanta." Then she asked, "Mr. Jones, have you tried to get an appointment at Emory?" "Ma'am," I said, "I want to be seen at the Mayo Clinic. I have been examined by most of the doctors around Atlanta and several other states, but the Mayo Clinic is where I want to be seen."

"Ok, Mr. Jones, but we need to know your main complaint," she replied. "Ma'am, I have a lot of them but since you asked what is my main complaint, let me tell you. I have been having prostate problems for 14 years. I can't get my asthma under control. My head is throbbing, I have diverticulitis. My back is always hurting. I'm in constant pain from four rotator cuff surgeries, two broken elbows and my vision is blurred," I explained.

"Mr. Jones it appears that you have a lot of problems, and I'm taking notes to assign you to a specialist for every body part that you have complained about," she said. She continued, "Mr. Jones, we have you on standby, and if an opening comes up, you need to accept the appointment because it's going to be hard or should I say it may take a long time for you to get another appointment. Also Mr. Jones, when we call, you should be prepared to stay in the area for three to five days. This is standard procedure just in case the doctors need you to report back to the clinic after they run tests." "Thank you Ma'am. I will be waiting for your call," I said.

A couple of weeks later I received a call from the Mayo Clinic asking me if I could report to their Clinic on October 18, 2010. "Yes Ma'am," I said, "I will be there." After I had gotten off the phone with the receptionist, I thanked God. However, on the inside of my heart, I was thinking after all these years, they were going to finally find out what was wrong with me. At least I will be up for the challenge to accept whatever they find. I knew God was going to work it out. He didn't allow me to get this far just to turn his back on me.

On October 18, 2010, I left Atlanta and arrived at the Mayo Clinic in Jacksonville, Florida at 5:30 a.m. I couldn't appreciate the ambience until daylight. The grounds were well manicured, and the Clinic reminded me of a college campus. They had two hotels on their campus, and everyone was so professional. I hoped that I would be seen quickly, but I was prepared to stay until I had gotten seen. I was a standby patient and was told that it was possible that I wouldn't be seen on the 18th, that it could be the next day. I called my publicist and lady friend in Orlando, Florida, to inform her as to what was going on, and I mentioned to her that I would be coming to stay with her after I was finished being examined at the Mayo Clinic. The time was 8:00 a.m. I had already registered at the front desk, hoping I would be seen if not that day maybe the next day.

CHAPTER 18

LET THE EXAMINATION BEGIN

The time was 8:15 a.m. Someone hollered, "Garry Jones!" "I'm Garry Jones," I replied. "Come with me," the nurse said. I got up and proceeded to follow the nurse to her office. "What brings you to the Mayo Clinic?" she asked. "Various things, but what I'm most concerned with is my prostate," I replied. "I'm looking over your notes, and notice that you have been having problems with your prostate for a long time," she stated. "Yes, I have. As a matter of fact, I started having problems with my prostate in 1998," I responded. "Do you have any other problems Mr. Jones?" the nurse asked. I replied, "I'm in the third stage of a chronic disease, asthma, four shoulder surgeries, two elbow surgeries, double hernia surgery, appendix removal, bullet removal, and I'm having a lot of headaches." The nurse said, "Mr. Jones, you are a good looking healthy man." "Thanks," I said, "but looks are deceiving."

"Where are you from," she asked. "I'm from Kinston, North Carolina," I responded. "Mr.

Jones, I studied at North Carolina State University in Raleigh, N. C.," she replied. "Oh you did," I said, "Well Laura, I studied at North Carolina Central University, and I'm sure you are familiar with N.C.C.U. considering we are located 26 miles apart." "Yes, Mr. Jones. I'm very familiar with that University," she said.

It had been two hours, and the nurse, who was an infectious disease specialist, and I had gone over my medical history. After she finished talking with me, she had accrued 12 pages of notes. "Mr. Jones, you came to the right place because whatever you have wrong with you we will find out," she informed me. "By the way Mr. Jones, how long are you going to be around the city?" she asked. "Laura, I'm going to be around the city as long as it takes. I'm retired, and I have only time on my hands," I responded. She continued, "Well today Mr. Jones, we are going to work you over for the next couple of days or possibly more. The only thing I have to do now is assign you to different specialists. They are going to examine you, and if they find anything wrong, you will be required to come back to the facility; that's why we ask our patients to be prepared to stay at least three days to a week."

"Where are you staying?" she asked. "Do you have relatives around the area?" "Yes,"

I said. "But I probably will be staying at a hotel, and I will be traveling to Orlando to see my lady friend." "I have children and friends in Tallahassee," I shared. The nurse continued, "Mr. Jones, the reason I have been talking to you ,taking notes, and putting them in the computer is because I'm trying to find out what openings are available for different specialists, today. During our time together and conversation, I have been completing an Infectious Disease Comprehensive History and Physical report." "Mr. Jones, are you ready for the examination to begin?" she inquired? "Laura, I was ready a couple of years ago," I replied. "Well Mr. Jones, here is your schedule, time and specialist to report to. This campus is big; it's just like being in college, and the doctors are your instructors," she stated. Laura concluded, "Mr. Jones, you probably won't see me again, but I will be checking on you to see how everything is going."

CHAPTER 19

MY MEDICAL WORKUPS

On the afternoon of October 18, 2010, all my lab work was done. I had the following examinations performed - a pathology report, EKG, Chest X-ray, and PFT's (Pulmonary Function Tests). My examinations were finish around 4:30 p.m. On October 19, 2010, I had a light day at the Mayo Clinic. I had a consultation with the Pulmonary Medicine Department. After my visit there, I got into my car and drove to Orlando, Florida to spend time with my lady friend. I didn't have to report back to the Mayo Clinic until October 28, 2010.

On the morning of October 28, 2010, my lady friend and I drove back to Jacksonville, Florida for my visit at the Mayo Clinic. This was the day that the doctor's would share my test results with me. I had the following examinations and consultations: CT Chest Hires. I met with the US Renal Department who checked for renal failure. I mentioned earlier that I was in the 3rd stage of a chronic kidney disease. I had a consultation with the

Polysomnography, which is a sleep specialist. I had a sleep study conducted later that night. This was unexpected, but an opening was available so I took the advantage of it.

It should be noted while you are at the Mayo Clinic an examination may be performed on you in the morning. Two hours later or the next day at the latest, the results are complete, unlike most doctors you visit. An examination and tests are conducted, and your results are ready within a week. Every test done at the Mayo Clinic is "stat", meaning the doctors want the test results within a couple of hours.

On October 29, 2010, I had a skin test conducted, and I had to undergo a Urology UFS. I had to void in a machine to test the stream flow of my urine.

Later on that day, I had an Allergy consultation, Sleep Consultation visit, and a consultation with the Urology Department. This consultation was very detailed and that was the way I wanted it. I didn't feel rushed, and the doctors were very concerned with what I had to say.

I was examined by two doctors, and this was their assessment:

10-29-2010 12:18p.m. EDT

SUPERVISING PHYSCIAN: Gregory Abbot, M.D.

REFERRING PHYSICIAN: Laura Campbell

CHIEF COMPLAINT

HISTORY OF PRESENT ILLNESS

Mr. Jones is a pleasant 46 year old gentleman who recently underwent Clinic Infectious Disease Comprehensive H&P on 10-18-2010. During that evaluation he had noted history of frequent urinary tract infections and a diagnosis of prostatitis, as well as microscopic hematuria. Urology consultation was requested.

Upon presentation today, Mr. Jones states that, approximately, 10 years ago he began having frequent urinary tract infections that he recalls being documented with urinalyses and cultures. They were treated successfully with antibiotics for duration but kept recurring. He has, for the past several years, been getting approximately 2 per year. He has been evaluated by an urologist, initially, about 8 years ago and been given a diagnosis of prostattitis. He has since seen several urologists and been on multiple courses of antibiotics for multiple durations, including for two weeks, for several months, and for up to a year.

Currently, he has prescriptions for ciprofloxacin and takes this when he begins having symptoms. His last symptomatic episode was approximately a year ago. He states when he has symptoms, he has high fever, lower back pain and dysuria. When he has these symptoms, he takes Cipro for 14 days and this usually alleviates his symptoms. He no longer follows up with any other urologist.

He does recall having flow studies but does not recall having CAT scans and does not recall being told there was anything abnormal with any imaging.

For the hematuria, he states he has never seen blood in his urine and was just told it was noted on urinalyses whenever he was symptomatic from infections. He does not recall ever being told he had microscopic hematuria without symptoms of urinary tract infections or prostatitis.

CHAPTER 20

ROUND 2 WITH THE SECOND UROLOGIST

I love how the doctors at the Mayo Clinic worked together. I didn't have to worry about getting a second opinion because after one doctor finished with me, they sent their notes to other doctors and conferred with them to get their opinion.

I left out of one Urologist's office and within an hour, I was in another Urologist office to get his opinion. Finally, someone was taking me seriously that I have been sick for 10 years.

Below is the FINAL REPORT and Findings:

This is a supervisory and confirmatory note for Brian Johnson, PA-C 1

Prior to interviewing and examine this patient, we reviewed a comprehensive history and physical examination performed by Laura Campbell, M.D.., on October 18, 2010. We reviewed current visit information and patient family history.

Mr. Brian Johnson has nicely documented the urologic history. This patient is referred with a chronic intermittent prostatitis. He has a rather complex medical history and is currently on numerous medications.

When asked whether or not the patient had trigger points for developing prostatitis, he stated maybe stress but the symptoms comes fast and before he knows it he is on the floor with flank pain. It seems that sexual activity, perineal compression or riding in a car or riding a bicycle has nothing to do with his intermittent prostatitis. The patient can recall taking the medication Nyquil and it trigger him to have another infection. Patient also said he can't tolerate spicy foods.

I have recommended an uroflow postvoid residual. If the patient is carrying residual or has depressed flow rates, then I would recommend a cystoscopy. His last cystoscopic examination was 2001.

To better assess the prostate, I think it would be reasonable to do an MRI at some time to rule out any evidence of prostatic abnormality prostatic abscess.

I had another appointment with one of three Urologists. The urologist stated that he wanted to do an MRI of my prostate area to rule out several things, mainly an abscess on the prostate. I was told the examination would be evasive but would not hurt. I agreed to have the procedure.

I shared with my lady friend what the doctors wanted to do next, and she seemed a little perplexed. I explained to her that they wanted to do an MRI of the prostate. She asked me when would the procedure be done, and I told her December 03, 2010. She recommended that we head back to Orlando to have some fun because the Mayo Clinic had worked me over. I informed my lady friend when we arrived back in Orlando that I wanted to take a helicopter ride so she suggested that we go on International Drive. I didn't have to report back to the Mayo Clinic until December 2, 2010. We returned to Orlando the next day, went down to International Drive, and took a helicopter ride over the city of Orlando.

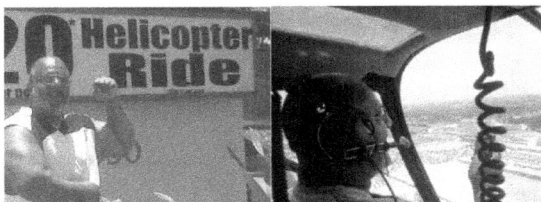

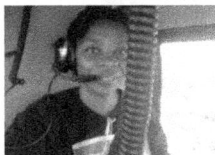

CHAPTER 21

RETURN VISIT TO THE MAYO CLINIC

On December 02, 2010, I returned to the Mayo Clinic for a series of test and test results. My schedule was hectic for that day and the following day. My lady friend accompanied me to all my appointments, like she always did. She had been there every step of the way. I could tell that she was concerned about what was going on. Today, my schedule was with the following specialists: MRI for the Brain, US DPlx Carotid, Neurology and Sleep Subsequent Visit.

My first appointment was the MRI (Magnetic Resonance Imaging) on the brain.

FINAL REPORT

CONCLUSION: There is no evidence for acute infarction on diffusion weighted images.

FINDINGS: No previous studies are available for comparison.

There is no evidence for acute infarction on diffusion weighted images. The ventricles and subarachnoid spaces are normal in size, shape, and position, without abnormal foci of increased or decreased signal intensity, focal intracranial mass lesion or mass effect in the brain parenchyma.

Incidental note is the presence of a complete or near complete mucosal pacification of the left frontal sinus with slight hyper intensity on T1, as well as marked hyper intensity on T2 and for images. This could represent inspissated secretions or a small mucocele.

The next appointment was with the US DPLX Carotid ATR. Department. In short the carotid artery is a major artery located in front of the neck. Through the carotid artery, blood from the heart goes to the brain. There are two common carotid arteries – the right and left common carotid arteries – one on each side of the neck.

FINAL REPORT

FINDINGS: Minimal endothelial thickening or plaque formation in both common carotid arteries distally. No appreciable plaque formation seen at the origin of internal or external arteries. Doppler wave forms and velocities are consistent with either no or minimal stenosis of the internal right arteries.

The next appointment was with the Nephrology Department for a consultation.

FINAL REPORT

Impression and Plan

STAGE III CHRONIC KIDNEY DISEASE. Mr. Jones gave a history of STAGE III chronic kidney disease for the last years or so and, according to him, his GFR (Glomular Filtration Rate) has been 53-54 ml/min and he had some proteinuria but no further treatment was given.

Review of the labs from here showed that his creatinine on October 18, 2010 was 1.4 and the urinalysis had trace proteinuria but it was fairly concentrated urine with a specific gravity of 1,023. His protein: creatinine ratio was less than 0.1 and micro albumin: creatinine ratio was in the normal range. His ultrasound showed 11.1 and 11.4 cm kidneys with mild increase echo texture of the kidney, It is possible that he had previous acute kidney injury in 2007 and had partial resolution of acute kidney injury with resultant CDK Chronic Kidney Disease) Also, he is a relatively obese person as well as has good muscle mass so a creatinine of 1.4 may not reflect a decrement of GFR for him. His urinalysis over here does not have significant proteinuria so, at this point based on the information available , it is not clear whether he really has STAGE III chronic kidney disease or not. At this point, I will recommend repeating his renal function panel and perform a 24-hour urine collection for creatinine and the protein to estimate his creatinine clearance and also to see the degree of proteinuria he has. He has a family history of renal failure but no history of hearing loss. He does not have a high grade proteinuria to consider familial focal segmental glomerulosclerosis as the etiology. It is likely that he may have underlying chronic tubular interstitial nephritis from-long standing use analgesics. We will also do the serologic workup to rule out autoimmune disease affecting the kidneys.

In conclusion other than what the doctor's assessed, it was great to have second opinions. *If you are not sure whether or not they have the right diagnosis, ask and ask again.* As you can see in the above reports, it was not determined whether or not I had STAGE III KIDNEY DISEASE, but the test results supported STAGE II KIDNEY DISEASE. Most patients are being misinformed on their diagnosis whether by sure ignorance of the doctor or purposefully for the purpose of putting them on medication to continue to make the pharmaceutical companies rich. It had been a long day so my lady friend/girlfriend and I headed back to the hotel. I had several more specialists to meet with the next day with the most important one being my Urology specialist.

CHAPTER 22

THE PROCEDURE I DREADED:
PELVIC MRI SCAN

On December 3, 2010 at 10:00 a.m., I had an appointment with my Orthopedic. His analysis indicated both my right and left rotator cuff in my shoulder were intact.

SHOULDER 4 VWS RT PLUS LT:

No comparison. Soft tissues anchor noted overlying humeral head for prior rotator cuff surgery. Glenohumeral articulation is well maintained. No tendentious calcification.

My next procedure was at 4:30 p.m. My doctor told me the procedure wouldn't hurt, but it would be uncomfortable. Most people wonder what a Pelvic M.R.I. is. Well, it's when a magnetic resonance imaging scan uses magnets and radio waves to capture images inside your body without making a surgical incision. The scan allows your doctor to see the soft tissues of the body, such as muscles, without your bones obstructing the view.

While an MRI can be done on any part of your body, a pelvic MRI scan specifically helps your doctor to see the bones, organs, blood vessels, and other tissues in your pelvic region- the area between your hips that holds your reproductive organs. This helps your doctor inspect potential problems found in other imaging tests, such as X-rays; diagnose unexplained hip pain; investigate the spread of certain cancers; or better understand the conditions causing your symptoms. It was amazing that I experienced joint and hip pain for many years. But because I was such an athlete, I blamed the pain on my age and the running that I used to do when I ran track.

Although the pelvic area holds your reproductive organs, your doctor may order the test for different reasons depending on if you are a male or female. The reason my doctor ordered the MRI for me was to investigate the urinary tract infections and to determine whether or not I had an abscess on my prostate. From this he could determine where the urinary tract infections were coming from. The doctors would use their findings to explain why I had been sick for so many years.

I was called to go in the examining room and asked whether or not I needed an anxiety pill. I told them that I take anxiety medication anyway. I had no a clue as to what would come next. After I took off my hospital gown, I was asked to get on the examining table and lie on my stomach. "Turn on my stomach. For what?" I asked. The technician informed me that he needed to put a metal rod (coil) in my rectum. "What the hell you just say?" I asked again. The technician replied, "Mr. Jones, that's how this procedure works, and after the metal is placed inside, then you go under the MRI machine." The technician proceeded to insert the metal rod into my rectum. "My doctor said it wasn't going to hurt but it is hurting," I said. "Mr. Jones, are you just uncomfortable or are you hurting?" the technician asked. "God dammit," I said, "I know the difference between uncomfortable and hurting. Go get my damn doctor." My doctor came in and asked, "What's going on, Mr. Jones?" "The metal rod that he has in my rectum is hurting," I said. The doctor looked at the technician in disgust and said, "The reason he is hurting is because the place where the rod is positioned is hitting on a bone." The doctor placed the metal coil in my rectum where it was supposed to be placed, and then I went under the MRI machine and went to sleep.

The technician tried to apologize to me, but I wouldn't accept his apology because he was trying to convince me I wasn't hurting;

he must have thought that I was a fool. I wasn't stupid. If that rod was not in my rectum, I probably would have gotten up and knocked the shit out of him.

CHAPTER 23

FINAL REPORT ON THE MRI PELVIC EXAM

REPORT WAS REVISED /RESENT TO ADD ORDERED PROCEDURE. REPORT CONTEXT UNCHANGED.

MR SPECTROSCOPY:

MR PELVIS WOW PLUS W/ CTS PLUS SED:

EXAM: Multiplanar imaging of the pelvis using the endorectal and surface coils, and including a volumetric spectroscopic spectroscopic acquisition. IV glucagon and 20 ml Omniscan per protocol.

CONCLUSION: Small spectroscopic abnormality in the posteror left peripheral zone, as detailed below. Recommend correlation with PSA.

FINDINGS: Mild central prostate hypertrophy. Otherwise, T2 diffusion, and perfusion weighted images show a normal appearing gland, with good zonal demarcation and peripheral zone (PZ) signal intensity. No evidence of imflamation, abscess, or fistula. However, on spectroscopy, there are 2 voxels with abnormal spectra at the junction of peripheral zone and central gland, left posterior base, less than 1cm from the midline. Despite the singularity of this finding, malignancy is to be excluded.

Seminal vesicles, rectum and bladder are unremarkable. No lymphadenopathy or other extraprostatic abnormality. Skeletal structures intact.

CHAPTER 24

GOD REVEALS PROSTATE CANCER

After the procedure was over my lady friend and I stayed in Jacksonville, Florida for a couple of days because I still had an appointment at the Mayo Clinic on December 6, 2010. After the appointment we, headed back to Orlando, Florida. When we arrived in Orlando, both of us were tired, and I was drained from being poked and prodded so many times. When I went to bed that night, I had one of the weirdest dreams. I dreamt that I was back in North Carolina. In the dream I woke up too late, and I told my grandmother I was running late for work even though I had already retired from work. My grandmother said that she was late for work too, and she was going to call in sick even though she didn't have a job. When I walked outside of my house, former Senator John Edwards was campaigning in front of my house. I saw one of my friends and went to the gym.

I awaken the next morning about 6:30 a.m. I asked myself, what was that dream all about. Around 10:30 a.m. I was looking at

CNN on television, and the news had broken about former Senator John Edwards's wife Elizabeth Edwards had passed away from cancer. After the news broke that was when I told my girlfriend about the dream. We were both sad about Mrs. Edwards succumbing to cancer. A couple of days later around December 12, 2010, my girlfriend and I went shopping. I had been in Orlando a long time, and I was headed back to Atlanta, Georgia. I received a call from the Mayo Clinic, and my doctor's assistant asked me whether or not I had gone back to Atlanta. I remembered telling her that I would be leaving to go back to Atlanta in a few hours.

She informed me that my doctor wanted me to come back to the Mayo Clinic. I asked her why, and she stated that my doctor wasn't comfortable with the pathology report on my Pelvis so he wanted me to return to the clinic to have a biopsy done. "When does the doctor want me to come back?" I asked. She said, "I can get you scheduled as soon as possible." The assistant then asked me to hold on for a second while she called the scheduling department. Shortly, she came back to the phone and told me that they could schedule me for the biopsy on December 15, 2010. I agreed and made plans to return to the Mayo Clinic on December 15, 2010.

I went back into one of the stores where my lady friend was shopping and informed her that I wasn't going back to Atlanta because the doctor's office had just called and wanted me to come back to the clinic to have a biopsy done. She asked me why. I played it off and said that they found a spot, and they just wanted to double check to make sure it wasn't cancer. I said, "You know how the Mayo Clinic is. They are real thorough." She was excited that I wasn't going back to Atlanta, but at the same time I could tell by the look on her face she was uneasy. I felt in my spirit that she knew that I knew why I was having the biopsy. We both knew what it was, but we didn't say it to each other. God had already warned me in my dream that I would be diagnosed with Prostate Cancer. There was a reason I dreamt about John Edwards only to find out the next day that his wife had died of cancer.

On December 15, 2010, my lady friend and I arrived back to the Mayo Clinic for my 11:00 a.m. appointment. "Garry Jones," the nurse said. "I am he," I responded. She asked, "What's your date of birth?" "January 25, 1964," I replied. "Mr. Jones, here is your gown," she said, "we need for you to undress and try to use the restroom. Once you finish Mr. Jones, just let us know, and you can follow us."

CHAPTER 25

THE PROCEDURE BEGINS

PREOPERATIVE DIAGNOSIS:

Elevated prostate-specific antigen

POST OPERATIVE DIAGNOSIS

Elevated prostate – specific antigen

PROCEDURE

1.   *Transrectal transonographic examination*

2.   *Transrectal ultrasound-guided prostate needle biopsies*

ANESTHETIC- LOCAL

SPECIMENS TO PATHOLOGY

Prostate cores

COMPLICATION

None

ESTIMATED BLOOD LOSS

Minimum.

PROCEDURE

The patient was brought into the Ultrasound Suite. The risks, goals, and complications related to prostate needle biopsy were reviewed with the patient: Specifically rectal pain, bleeding, infection, acute urinary retention, or hematuria.

Thereafter, the patient was placed on the examination table in the lateral decubitus position. Lidocaine anesthetic was in infiltrated into the perirectal tissues manually. Following this, the 7.5 MHz B&K ultrasound scanner was introduced into the rectum. Imaging of the prostate was conducted from the base to the apex. The patient tolerated the procedure well. The patient was given antibiotic prophhylaxis.

When the doctor was doing the biopsy, he had a conversation with the nurse. He slipped and said "I thought the cancer was on the left side of the prostate." I immediately asked, "Are you telling me that I have Prostate cancer?" as if I didn't already know. The doctor stated that they had to wait for the results of the biopsy to give a definitive answer.

FINDING

Volumetric assessment was performed; 32.8 gm of tissues were noted. Also noted were hypoechoic changes to the left peripheral zone. Ten core biopsies were performed and sent to pathologic review. These consisted of anterior horn biopsy 1, anterior horn biopsy 2, base, mid, apex. Those were repeated on the right and the left

Procedure was well tolerated. Patient had minimal hemorrhage. Antibiotic prophylaxis was administered given his history of prostatits.

After the procedure was conducted, my lady friend and I went to St. Augustine, Florida to shop. I purchased my lady friend and my sister a gift. After a while the anesthesia began to wear off, and I started to feel a lot of pain in my rectum. I purchased some Tylenol Extra Strength, but it wasn't working. I went to the restroom, and urinated out a lot of blood. This was no surprise because I was told in advance that this may happen over the next three months. I couldn't deal with the pain so I called my doctor, but he wasn't available. I spoke with his nurse, and she asked if I had a pharmacy that I used in Orlando. She called in some powerful pain medication for me. I was miserable, and I was not in the holiday spirit. I was trying not to complain because I wanted my lady friend's spirit to continue to be uplifted.

When we arrived in Orlando, the only thing that I wanted to do was rest. The blood in the urine lasted only for a couple of months. I was planning on leaving to go back to Atlanta, Georgia the next day but I didn't feel up to it so I laid around for a couple of days until I could regain my energy.

CHAPTER 26

RECEIVED THE BAD NEWS WHILE DRIVING

As soon as I got enough energy to travel, I went back to Atlanta. It was December 23rd when I left Orlando, Florida. I was trying to get back to Atlanta to catch a flight out on December 24th to go home to Kinston, N. C. for the holidays. Prior to me leaving, I called the Mayo Clinic to get the results of my biopsy, but the doctor wasn't in. A few hours later the phone rang. I said, "Hello." The voice on the other end said, "May I speak with Garry Jones?" I said, "This is he." "Mr. Jones, this is your doctor. Have you departed the Florida area?" he asked. I answered, "Yes." He asked, "Are you sitting down?" I said, "Yes, I'm sitting down and going about 80 miles per hours." "Mr. Jones is there any way that you could pull to the side of the road where we can talk," the doctor asked. I said, "No, whatever information you have to tell me, you can tell me now while I'm riding."

"Mr. Jones, it's not common practice that I speak to my patients on the phone regarding their medical condition, but considering you are on your way back to Atlanta, will it be ok for me to tell you what the Biopsy revealed," he said. "Sir, with all due respect, I know what the biopsy revealed. I know I have prostate cancer," I said. "Mr. Jones, you are correct," the doctor said, "and Mr. Jones, I don't want to ruin your holidays, but I do want to get you back in my office so we can discuss how we are going to attack this disease." "Mr. Jones, you are a healthy young man, and you have time on your side," the doctor continued, "and I suggest we remove your prostate." "But I want you to think about it, and I want to send you to doctors to discuss other options such as radiation and chemotherapy." "Mr. Jones, if you were an older man, I wouldn't recommend that you have your prostate removed," the doctor said. "If you prefer, you can consider 'watchful waiting'," he said. "I asked, "What is that?" He said, "In six months we can do another biopsy to determine whether or not the tumor is getting bigger. But considering your history of urinary tract infections, we may need to take action sooner." "Mr. Jones, I don't want you to worry, but I do want you to have a Merry Christmas," he said. "Dr. Bill, I'm not worried at all," I said, "as a matter of fact, I feel good because it's over. For all the years I had known that I was sick, and now that you all have discovered what my illness is, the world has been lifted off of my shoulder." After I got off the phone with the doctor, I continued to drive without a worry in the world. I called my lady friend and gave her the news; she was quiet.

When I arrived in Atlanta, I repacked my luggage and headed for North Carolina the very next day. My Christmas was great. I called my pastor and informed him what was going on, and he prayed for me on the phone. He asked me whether or not they had found the cancer in time, and I told him that I thought so. I discussed my medical situation and diagnosis with my family in North Carolina. We all celebrated Christmas. I called my children in Tallahassee to let them know that their father was diagnosed with Prostate cancer. They all took it very well because to them it appeared that it didn't bother me, and they knew their daddy was a fighter. They had witness this first hand. I was ready to get back to Atlanta because I had concert tickets to see Tina Marie and

Maze featuring Frankie Beverly on New Year Day. I turned on the news, and heard that Tina Marie was found dead by her daughter on December 27, 2010.

CHAPTER 27

CONFIRMATION LETTER FROM THE DOCTOR

On December 30, I flew back to Atlanta, and I had already forgotten that I had prostate cancer because I was shocked by Tina Marie's death. Thank God I had already seen her perform with Rick James. On December 31, 2010, I went to Liberation Eve Services at our church to bring in the 2011 New Year. I had a great time at church, but I looked forward to seeing the big show, Maze and Frankie Beverly's performance. I didn't have a clue as to who was going to open for Maze. Later on that evening, I asked my cousin Ann was she ready to go to the show, and she said that she was.

I was excited although I had seen Maze and Frankie Beverly perform over 40 times. Each time I went I felt as though it was my first time seeing the group's performance. Ann and I went to our seats and mind you, we were only 13 rows from the stage. The show started and Johnny Gill came onto stage and rocked the house for twenty minutes. Ten minutes later the legendary Stephanie Mills came on the stage and turned it out. I was having the best time of my life.

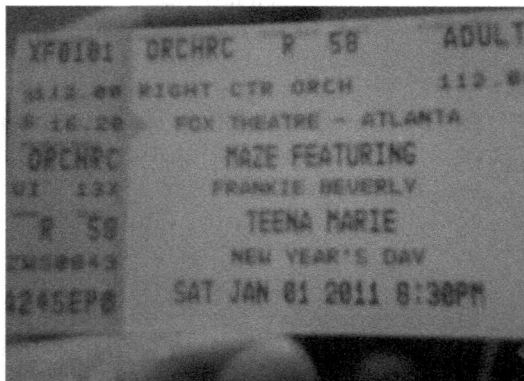

Tickets to Maze Featuring Frankie Beverly/Teena Marie Concert

An hour later the main act came on stage, and it was on and popping. Everyone stood up for the first 10 minutes when Maze and Frankie Beverly came on stage. After the first two songs, Frankie stopped the show and said, "This is a celebration of what Tina Marie would have loved." "Now let's tear the roof off of this place!" The Foxx Theater hadn't been the same since that show. Little did I know 24 days later, I would be on my death bed.

A couple of days later, I received a letter from my doctor confirming the conversation we had on the phone regarding the prostate.

The Letter:

Dear Mr. Jones:

I am writing you this brief letter to include copies of your workup here at the Mayo Clinic, including your recent pathology report.

I note from your chart that in my absence Eric Koonce, P.A.C.; informed you that the biopsy performed here at the Mayo Clinic have shown a single focus of prostate cancer.

As you will remember, your workup here at the Mayo Clinic was motivated by your history of intermittent prostatits. As part of that workup, I performed or requested a magnetic resonance imaging (MRI) to be performed on December 03, 2010. The MRI did not show us any evidence of prostate abscess, but did suggest an abnormal signal was coming from your prostate. The subsequent biopsy performed on December 15, 2010, has shown a single focus of prostate cancer, which is a very favorable Gleason score and shows a very small amount of cancer at that.

I would like to see you back as soon as we can discuss with you management of this newly diagnosed prostate cancer. For a man in your young age group, I generally recommend surgical removal of the prostate.

Alternatively, because it is such a small volume of disease, an argument could be made for a short period of watchful waiting to see whether or not this cancer is becoming clinically significant. That would require a serial prostate-specific antigen (PSA) drawn in three to four months and a repeat prostate needle biopsy in six months.

My office will be contacting you to schedule an appointment to sit down and discuss with me the pathology report and to meet one of my colleagues who does robotic radical prostatectomy.

CHAPTER 28

CONSULTATION FOR SURGERY

The next week I took a plane to Orlando, Florida, to meet with my lady friend before I went to Jacksonville, Florida to the Mayo Clinic for the consultation.

On the morning of January 17, 2011, I had an appointment with Dr. Ted to discuss the surgery. After we discussed the surgery he sent out a final report.

Please see the excellently detailed Urology consult of Gregory Brown, M.D. ; from 10/29/2010, as well as Urology prostate note from 12/15/2010, and urology notes from Eric Koonce , P.A.C.; on 12/20/2010.

For past medical history, past surgical history, medications, allergies Family history, social history, and complete review of systems, please see Brian Johnson's excellently detailed 10/29/2010 Urology consult.

PHYSICAL EXAMINATION

ABDOMEN: Soft. He has an exploratory laparotomy incision from a gunshot wound. He also has a laparoscopic hernia with mesh.

This is a 46 year old black male who has had 10 episodes of recurrent prostatitis, going 3 times per year. He requires antibiotics for this. He said it made his life miserable. Dr. Brooks saw the patient for this and did an MRI, which found prostate cancer by MRI findings. Prostate biopsy revealed a Gleason 6 adenocarinoma, 5% of 1 core. His PSA is very low; it is under 1.

His SHIM score is 13. His AUA score with a 10 with the problem of chronic prostatitis as I mentioned previously.

Discussed issues with Mr. Jones. I discussed that he could do watchful waiting. The problem with that is his young age. He does not want to do that. He also does not want to do radiation, as he has done his research and knows that there are problems with his recurrent prostatitis and radiation.

He wants the surgery. He wants robotic surgery. He has been told that he needs prostatectomy. He is very interested in robotic surgery. The robotic surgery

112

poses for him is exploratory for a laparotomy for a gunshot wound, and appendectomy. He also has laparoscopic hernia with mesh. He has an incision in the sub umbilical region. I think we can get abdominal access. I told him that there is a possibility we may have a bowel injury, If that is the case, he may require conversion to an open operation or open prostatectomy, as well as possibly even colostomy. Discussed the risk of rectal injury during the surgery that may require colostomy. I want to try abdominal access in him. I think we can do it.

Discussed prostatectomy in great detail, and I drew pictures of the operation. Discussed risk of infection. Discussed risk of prolonged catheterization for non-healing anastomosis.

Discussed the risk of urinary incontinence while in surgery. Discussed low SHIM score; there is a high likelihood he would not have spontaneous erections after surgery. Discussed risk of major vascular incident during surgery including but not proceed with robotic prostatectomy and possible conversion to an open operation. I am going to ask him to wait a few months after his prostate biopsy given the problems he has had with urgency, frequency, and prostatitis.

Will give him the antibiotics about 10 days before the surgery to try and cut down any risk of inflammation of prostatitis.

The doctor and I agreed that the surgery would take place on March 9, 2011. I understood that I may have complications during the surgery. It must be noted that after they scheduled me for surgery, and I began to consider the complications that I may have because of my medical history, I changed my mind about having the surgery. I didn't let anyone know that I had decided that right before the surgery was to take place, I was going to pull out. I knew I wasn't going to be able to produce another child, and I was with a woman who didn't have any children.   As soon as accepted my decision of not going through with the surgery, God intervened. And what happen next convinced me to have the surgery.

CHAPTER 29

I WAS DYING AND DIDN'T KNOW IT

It was two days before my birthday on January 23, 2011. I was in Orlando, Florida, chilling with my lady friend. I called a couple of friends in Tallahassee that were all pumped for the AFC (American Football Conference) Championship game between the Pittsburg Steelers and the New York Jets. We were all talking on the phone on 3-way. The game aired at 6:30 p.m. eastern standard time. It didn't matter to me who won the game because I had already booked my flight, hotel room, and rental car to fly to Dallas, Texas for Super Bowl XLV to be played in the Dallas Cowboys Stadium on February 06, 2011. Let me retract. It did matter to me who won the game, and I wasn't pulling for Pittsburg. One of my friends was a stone cold, diehard Steeler's fan, and the other friend was from Houston, and she could have cared less about who won the game.

The only thing I knew was that we were laughing and joking on the phone. I even had a couple of beers. The Pittsburg Steelers won the game 24-19 and was going to the Super Bowl to play the Green Bay Packers who had beaten the Chicago Bears earlier in the NFC (National Football Conference). After the game was over, I made a couple of contacts with people whom I knew that would give me a reasonable price for tickets for the Super Bowl game. I remembered going to bed happy that Sunday night. My birthday was in two days, and I was going to the Super Bowl. I needed to have a good time, but my mind was still set on calling off the surgery to remove my prostate schedule for March 9, 2011.

Later on that night I was awaken from my sleep because of tremendous pain. I went to the bathroom, and I was burning so bad. It felt as though someone had cut my penis with a razor blade and poured alcohol all over it, again. I already knew what was going on. Yes, I had another urinary tract infection. I shook my head and said, "Damn, this is the twenty-first urinary tract infection in a matter of 10 years." I took a shower and went in the bedroom. I put on my sweat pants and went and sat in the living room; waiting for day light. It was around 3:30 a.m. My lady friend got up and came in the living room and asked me whether or not I was going walking. She thought it was about 6:30 a.m. I told her no because I was sick again, and I didn't want to go to the emergency room just to wait forever. I just wanted to go to Urgent Care to get some antibiotics and some pain medication. I thought maybe I would feel better by mid-afternoon when the medication began to take effect.

Unfortunately, Urgent Care was not accepting any patients so I was forced to go to the emergency room. My lady friend drove me to the hospital, and I waited for two hours before they called me in the back. When the doctors asked me what was going on I told them that I had a urinary tract infection. They asked me how I knew. I told them this was my twenty-first infection, and I was quite familiar with the routine. When they took my urine and a culture, they realized that my personal diagnosis had proven to be correct. I asked them to give me some antibiotics and pain pills. They prescribed the antibiotic Cipro, and I don't remember what pain medication they prescribed. My lady friend and I left the hospital. While I lay in bed, my lady friend went to get my

117

prescription filled, and I also asked her to get me soup and Ginger Ale while she was out. This was the day before my birthday, and I wanted to make sure that I felt better on my birthday. My condition began to get worse. I was in so much pain that my head was throbbing, my temperature was around 103, my back was hurting, and all my bones were aching. I could barely see. I thought to myself that this was not an ordinary urinary tract infection. I kept throwing up all over the place. I couldn't get any relief from the pain although I was taking the pain medication. I told my lady friend to go back out and get me something stronger than Ginger Ale and to bring me some more soup back, maybe I could keep that down in my stomach. When she came back to the apartment, I was on the floor in the bedroom in a fetal position. She helped me get back in bed, but I wasn't comfortable in the bed. I ate the soup and vomited it back up.

The time was around 4:00 p.m., and I asked my lady friend, "What hospital did they take Tiger Woods to when he and his wife had been fighting about his indiscretion?" She said, "They took him to Health Central." I then said, "Take me there." When she got herself together and was ready to go, I had changed my mind about going to the hospital. I felt as though I was losing my mind because I was in so much pain. She asked me if I wanted to go to the hospital via the ambulance, and I told her no because an ambulance would bring on too much attention. The fact that I didn't go to the hospital by ambulance was probably one of the worse mistakes that I could have ever made. Around 6:00 p.m. she took me to Health Central, and everybody and their mother was in the waiting room. I was checked in at the front desk and was told to have a seat. I couldn't get comfortable. One time I was in a wheel chair, and then I was in a fetal position on the floor in the emergency room. I kept returning to the front desk asking what was taking so long.

I asked the secretary at the front desk to give me a cup so that I could urinate in and she asked why. I told her it was because when the doctors call me back, I wanted them to have the results of my urine test ready. The doctors finally called me back around 10:30 p.m. and put me in a room. I was begging for water or some ice to suck on, but they refused. I asked them to go ahead and get me some pain medication. The truth, as I remember, was that I was stuck with a needle 12 times that night, and they couldn't draw any blood. To make matters worse, they couldn't alleviate my pain because they couldn't get an I.V. inserted into my hand. I kept asking my lady friend the time because I didn't want my birthday to start at the hospital. One of the nurses came in and started hooking me up to a heart monitor. I told her there was nothing wrong with my heart. The doctor came in and looked at the heart monitor, and I asked why was hooked to a heart monitor machine. The doctor ignored me and walked out of the room. I became pissed and demanded the nurse go back and get the doctor so that he could tell me what was wrong. Hell, I knew that I had a urinary tract infection and the nurse confirmed that. I asked the nurse what was going on, and she said that the doctor had to share that information with me. When the doctor came back in the room, he said I had congestive heart failure.

The doctor left again, and I asked the nurse to go get the doctor because I needed more information about my condition. When the doctor returned to the room, I shared with the doctor everything that was going on with my body. He said, "Mr. Jones your organs are shutting down." I said, "Ok, fix it, but give me something for my pain and get the organs back to normal so I can go." It was almost 12:00 midnight, and I wanted to be out of that hospital before my birthday. The doctors looked at me and said that there wasn't too much that they could do when the body's organs start to shut down. He said that my kidneys were shutting down and so was my liver. I said, "Like I said before, get them back to normal." The doctor said, "Mr. Jones, we are afraid that maybe a cancer cell has gotten out, has gone through the blood stream, and started shutting your organs down." I said, "Ok." He said, "Mr. Jones, when your organs shut down you die. We are running tests because all the antibiotics that you are taking are not working, and we have to do a culture to see which antibiotics your body will accept." "We should know something in 24 hours that will help us to identify what will work for you," he continued. The doctor walked out of the room, and the nurse came in and finally was able to insert an IV in my hand to get the pain medication into my system. I asked, "Vikki (lady friend), what time is it? I'm ready to go home." She said, "It's around 11:30 p.m." The nurse interject and said, "Mr. Jones, you are not going home; you are being admitted." When the clock struck 12, it was my birthday, and I was mad as hell. I was being rolled upstairs in a hospital room. I said, "Vikki call my Aunt Colleen and tell them what's going on. And tomorrow call my children and let them know what is going on, as well."

The nurse came in the room and administered something into my I.V. to help relieve my pain and put me to sleep, but I started feeling hot all over. I asked the nurse, "What in the hell did you just give me?" She replied, "Morphine." I told the nurse to get that morphine out of me. I didn't know morphine made people feel like that. I began to feel anxious. Somehow they were able to reverse the morphine and give me another pain medication. I went to sleep for a couple of hours, and when I awaken, Vikki was doing her homework. She didn't sleep at all. She left the room for a couple of hours and brought me back a birthday gift.

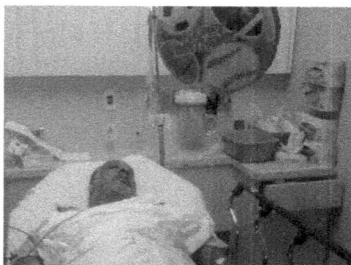

When I Initially Arrived to Health Central

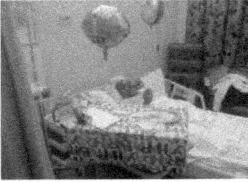
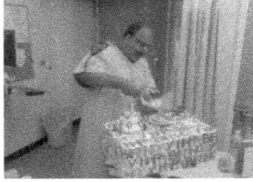
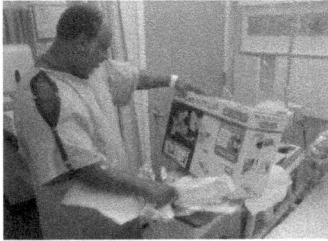

My Birthday from Vikki
Is she telling me that I need to lose the stomach?

The doctors came in and said, "Mr. Jones, we have already scheduled a kidney specialist and a liver specialist to examine you. You are still in bad shape." I said, "That's fine. I need to be out of here by Wednesday because I have a plane to catch. I'm going to the Super Bowl." The doctor said, "Mr. Jones, you won't be going to the Super Bowl, and hopefully when the culture comes back, we can determine if there is an antibiotic to fight the infection in the body."

I was angry as hell. I was in the hospital on my birthday and now they were telling me that I couldn't go to the Super Bowl. On January 27, 2011, I received a call from my brother Pete and Shellcat, my Super Bowl travelers. My brother Pete said, "You can do all the faking you want to do, but you are not going to get your share of the hotel money and car rental money back so you had better get well and catch your flight to Dallas to join us for the Super Bowl." The doctors came in and said, "Mr. Jones, we think we have found an antibiotic to fight the infections in your body. I will have my nurse administer this to you right away." I was still pissed off at my brother. An hour later a friend of the family arrived to visit me, with her scared self. Patricia was just like an aunt. She and my aunt Denderant were the best of friends, and Patricia treated my brother and me like we were her nephews. She was nervous as hell. She said she didn't like to be around sick people, and I told he that I didn't like being sick. A few minutes later I got up to go to the bathroom. When I came back to my bed, I didn't have any oxygen. The nurse and the doctors rushed in and immediately wanted to rush me to intensive care.

While they were waiting for an intensive care bed, I had to find a way to get my oxygen back because I didn't want to die. The staff administered oxygen to me, and my oxygen levels began to rise. I still wasn't out of the woods. All of a sudden, I had an epiphany. I realized that I was really, really sick. When the doctors started to administer the new antibiotics, my kidney levels and liver levels began to rise but not to the point that I was stable. A couple of days later, the Super Bowl game came on, and I had to watch the Super Bowl in the hospital. On February 08, 2011, I was released from the hospital. I had some time to myself to chat with God, and I realized that he allowed me to get sick because He knew that I needed to go ahead with the surgery.

CHAPTER 30

THE TIME ARRIVED TO REMOVE THE PROSTATE

After being in the hospital for eight days a couple of months prior and one step away from death, I was convinced God was giving me a second chance for my life to be saved. On paper it appeared that my cancer was small, but it was giving me big time problems. It was as though I could hear God talking to me saying, "Goldwater, for years you wanted to know what was going on with your health, having infection after infection- twenty-one to be exact. Now that you know that you have prostate cancer, you want to change your mind about having the surgery. I kept Satan from taking your life by preventing the cancer cells from getting into your blood stream and shutting your organs down. My child, I had to allow you to experience what could have happen if your organs had shut down." I heard God say, "My child the procedure you are going to go through is not an easy procedure, but I will give the doctors a plan to handle any complications because the area of your body that they need to maneuver through will be problematic because of your past surgeries. I assure you they will not have to cut you open."

The day prior to the surgery was very quiet between me and my lady friend. She was nervous, but I wasn't. I had been operated on at least 11 times, and I wasn't afraid. The only concern that I had was whether or not I would experience incontinence and for how long. Incontinence is the uncontrollable loss of urine or stool that is large or frequent enough to cause a social or health problem. It is a problem that can be very upsetting and embarrassing. But many people don't discuss the situation with their doctors, despite the fact that 80% of urinary incontinence cases can be cured or improved.

I had been doing the Kegel exercises for weeks to eliminate experiencing a lot of incontinence after the surgery. If you practice Kegel exercises, also called pelvic floor exercises, for five minutes, two or three times daily, you will likely see significant improvement in your ability to control urinary leakage. Another bonus: Kegel exercises can also help you have more intense orgasms and improve erections.

My lady friend and I left from Orlando, Florida, around 2:00 p.m. on March 8, 2011, and drove to Jacksonville, Florida where the Mayo Clinic was located. We checked in a hotel and went to get her something to eat. I couldn't eat anything because I was on a liquid diet. My cousin Ann had called and asked me if I was ok, and I said that I was fine. I hadn't heard from my brother nor my children. I knew my brother was flying in from North Carolina, and I knew my children and grandchildren, Derrick, LaToya, Malcolm, Derion and Jada were coming from Tallahassee. My youngest son Malcolm drove to Atlanta to catch a ride with his brother and sister. Nevertheless, I hadn't heard from them. I really didn't want any family members changing their schedule to be with me. I knew I was going to be fine.

After my lady friend Vikki had gotten her something to eat we both went back to the hotel. She was quiet, and I could tell she was nervous. I was wondering what was going through her mind. I wondered was she thinking that I didn't give her a baby because she knew after the surgery I wasn't going to be able to produce any more children. Did she think that I had cheated her out of a child? Well, I didn't want to bring another child in this world at the age of 47, knowing that I wasn't financially stable. I knew I wasn't going to have the patience and the energy to raise a child like I raised my other children. Hopefully, she wasn't thinking this way, but if she was, she had every right to.

I had to be at the Mayo Clinic at 5:00 am the next morning. On the morning of March 9, 2011, we drove across town to the Mayo Clinic and arrived around 4:55 a.m. Vikki went to park the car, and I went to the front desk to check in. I met this kid from another country, I can't recall exactly where from, but he had already had three surgeries for the problems he was having. He could barely speak English, but we were able to communicate. The young kid was nervous, and I gave have him a pep talk. Vikki came in, and the nurse came out and said, "Mr. Jones, you and your wife follow me." She didn't know that Vikki wasn't my wife, and I didn't correct her. After we arrived on the fifth floor and checked in, they gave me an instrument that lit up when the surgery team was ready for me. When the instrument lit up, the nurse called my name. I gave Vikki my things, kissed her and went back to the operating room. I thought to myself, if anything happens that I wasn't expecting, Vikki's face would have been the last face that I saw alive because neither my children nor brother had arrived.

When I arrived in the preparation room the doctors took my vitals and asked whether or not I was alright, and I told them yes. "Mr. Jones, do you need anything to calm you down?" they asked. "No I don't," I said. "Mr. Jones, we usually give the patients anxiety medication before we transport them back for surgery," the doctors stated. I said, "If that is your procedure, then go ahead and administer the medication through my veins."

CHAPTER 31

ON MY WAY TO THE OPERATING
ROOM

When I arrived in the operating room, I saw a team of five or six doctors. "Mr. Jones, how you feel?" they asked. "I feel fine," I replied. "Mr. Jones, we are going to put foam under your body so we can transfer you to the operating table," they said. I asked, "Are you all that strong?" They started laughing. I said, "As a matter of fact, I can easily slide myself onto the table." They said that they needed to assist and were surprised that I used my own strength to get onto the table. I looked at the doctors and told them that they looked nervous. They all started laughing. I broke out with a song by Maze and Frankie Beverly "Joy and Pain." The doctors asked me who sang the song. I said, "You don't anything about Frankie Beverly," and by the way "Why are you all taking so long to get started?" They said, "We are waiting for your doctor to arrive." "You know he is the best doctor in the world who does the Robotic surgery, so I heard," I said. When my doctor arrived, the surgery went as followed:

PROCEDURE

1.   *Laparoscopy with lysis of adhesions.*

2.   *Robotic-assisted laparoscopic prostatectomy bilateral athermal nerve sparing).*

FINAL REVIEWER AND ATTENDING PHYSCIAN

DAVID West, M.D.

PROCEDURE

After proper consent was obtained and the patient identified as Garry Jones, he was brought into the operating room and placed in the supine position, at which time general anesthesia was administered, and orogastric tube was placed. The patient was then placed in the dorsal lithotomy position using Allen stirrups, with care taken to cushion all pressure points, including ankles, knees, hips, wrist and elbows, His arms were tucked to his side in standard fashion. His chest was taped to the table over the foam padding to prevent slippage during steep Trendelenburg position. The patient's abdomen, penis, and perineum were sterilely prepped and draped in the standard sterile fashion.

He had a previous exploratory laparotomy incision for a gunshot wound. He also had bilateral hernias with mesh. We made a supraumbilical incision down to his fascia. The fascia was incised. The peritoneum was incised. His abdomen was entered. There was a minor amount of adhesion that was cut away. No bowel violation was noted during this step. A 12mm trocar was placed in, and the abdomen was inflated. We were able to see an area to get the 8mm, left-sided robotic port in 15 cm from the mid-portion of the pubic bone and 8 m from the midline. Adhesion (Scar Tissue) was cut away. No bowel violation was noted. Am 8 mm robotic port was placed 10 cm lateral to the left-sided 8 mm robotic port. An 8 mm robotic port was placed 15 cm from the mid-portion of the pubic bone and 8 cm from the midline on the right side, A 12 mm assistant port was placed 7 cm superolateral to the right-side 8 mm robotic port. A 5 mm assistant port was placed 7 cm superolateral to the 12 mm supraumbilical camera port. Inspection of the abdomen revealed no bowel violation. We later inspected the abdomen following specimen removal *after prostatectomy and again noted no bowel violation. The adhesions had been meticulously taken down.*

The patient was placed in steep Trendelenburg position, and the robot was docked in the standard fashion.

The bladder was taken down by incising lateral to the obliterating umbilical ligaments. He had a bilateral hernias with mesh. There was some adhesion in this area. Regardless, we were able to dissect the space of Retzius and free the pubic bone of its attachments. Fat overlying the prostate and enddopelvic fascia was removed. The superficial dorsal vein was sacrificed with bipolar cautery and monopolar cutting. .

The endoplevic fascia was incised on the right and left hands sides of the prostate, and levator ani muscles were teased away from the prostate up to the apex of the prostate. The dorsal vein was circumferentially dissected free of its attachments and secured with a #0 Vicryl stitch on a CT1 needle.

With a 30 degree downward-facing lens in place, the anterior bladder neck was opened. The previously-placed 22-French catheter balloon was taken down, and the catheter was elevated superiorly to give good retraction of the prostate. The posterior prostate was separated from the bladder neck. The seminal vesicles and vas deferens were identified and elevated in the standard fashion and dissected free of their attachments in the standard fashion. Sharp cutting was used to incise Denonvilliers fascia. I believe because of the patient's previous prostatitis, this area had a lot of adhesion and was very sticky. Regardless, we did meticulous dissection between the prostate and the rectum, and a safe plane was created.

Bilateral athemal nerve sparing ensued in the standard fashion. The lateral prostatic fascia was incised on the right- and left-hand sides of the prostate and teased away from the side of the prostate. This was also tedious because of what I believe was his previous prostatitis. There was a lot of inflammation in this area. The prostatic pedicles were secured with Weck clips. The prostatic pedicles were later oversewn with 3-o VICRYL and RB-1 needles for any active bleeders that existed.

With a catheter in the urethra and a 0-degree lens placed, the apex of the prostate was cut. The rectourethrails muscle was cut, and the prostate was *freely mobile and placed in a Endocatch bag. Inspection of the rectum revealed no violation. A 14-French red rubber catheter was placed in the rectum, and with fluid in the pelvis, air was injected into the catheter. No air bubbles were noted in the abdomen. Direct rectal examination revealed no palpable. Abnormality. And no blood on the glove.*

Urethrovesical anastomosis was completed with double-armed, 2-0 Monocryl on SH needles from 6 o'clock to 12 o'clock in a running Van Velthoven-type fashion, with the knot tied to 12 o'clock. A final 20-French catheter was placed in the bladder, with 20 ml in the balloon. The catheter was irrigated with 120 ml of normal saline. No extravasation was noted. Note that before anastomosis was completed, indigo carmine was given intravenously and noted to be effluxing from both ureteral orifices.

The prostate and its Endo Catch bag were removed by extending the 12 mm supraumbilical site. The fascia was closed with interrupted #1 PDS in a figure-of-eight fashion. All laparoscopic ports were removed under direct vision. No active bleeding was noted. A J-P drain was placed in the pelvis and anchored to the skin with silk suture. A final review of the abdomen revealed no active bleeding. There was no small bowel or large bowel violation that was evident.

All skin and port sites were closed with 4-0 Monocryl in a running subcuticular fashion. The Patient tolerated the procedure well.

When I opened my eyes, I asked the doctor were they able to save the nerve that causes erection, and they said yes. They didn't have any problems in that area. Vikki was next to my side, and she walked out with the doctor when they took me out of the recovery room to my own room. I spotted my children, my grandchildren, and my brother. They asked me if I was alright, and I told them that I was fine, and the doctors were able to save the nerve that causes an erection. I felt damn good. I hated wearing that catheter, though.

A couple of hours later, I was in the hallway walking, although I didn't feel up to walking. I was agitated that I had to wear that catheter. My brother had taken my children out to eat, and when they returned to the room, they stayed a couple more hours but then had to leave. A little later my brother had to leave, but he said that he would come back and see me in the morning.

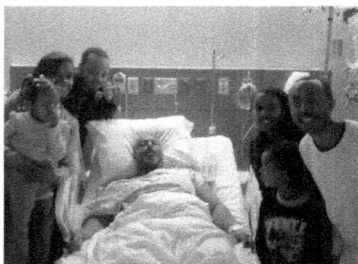

After Surgery with My Children
Derrick, Sherri, Dereon, Malcolm, LaToya, and Jada

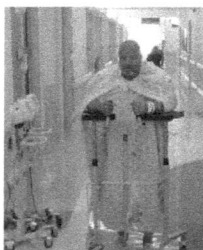

Walking in Hallways

CHAPTER 32

DISCHARGED: DIAGNOSIS REPORT

I was discharged from the Mayo Clinic on March 11, 2011.

DISCHARGED DIAGNOSIS

PROSTATE CANCER

HOSPITAL COURSE

COMORBID DIAGNOSIS

1.   OBSTRUCTIVE SLEEP APNEA

2.   AORTIC REGURGITATION

3.   CHRONIC KIDNEY DISEASE

Mr. Jones is a 47 year old- gentlemen diagnosed with Gleason 3+3 = 6 adenocarinoma on December 15, 2010. He underwent Da Vinci Robotic prostatectomy with David West, M.D.; on March 09, 2011. For full operative note, please see Power Chart. The patient was brought up to the 5th floor with no complications.

On Postoperative day 1, there were no acute events overnight. No complaints of chest pains, shortness of breath, or nausea or vomiting. He was tolerating a clear liquid diet, and his pain was under control. His abdomen was soft, nondistended with appropriate postoperative tenderness. JP was draining a small amount of serosanguineous fluids and his Foley catheter was place draining pink urine. His hemoglobin 12.5, hematocrit 37.3, creatinine 1.4.which is stable for him. He is afebrile. Vital signs are stable and adequate urine output. Later on that afternoon he was tolerating a regular diet and ambulating the halls.

On postoperative day 2, there was no acute event overnight. His pain was under control with just p.o. medication. He was tolerating a regular diet and ambulating the hall. His abdomen was soft, non-distended. He had appropriate postoperative tenderness. His JP drain was removed. Foley catheter remained in place draining clear urine. His vital signs were stable and he was afebrile with adequate urine output. He was deemed ready for discharge.

FOLLOWUP APPOINTMENT

The patient will be seen in the clinic on Wednesday, March 16, 2011 for Foley catheter removal.

I hated leaving the hospital with that catheter on especially since I had to wear it for one week.

Vikki and I checked into a hotel room nearby because the doctors wanted me to be close just in case of an emergency. The first day I wanted to rest, but Vikki wanted me to walk around the hotel to get some exercise. I didn't have a problem with the exercise, it was more that I didn't like walking with a catheter. I had to wear long sweat pants to hide the catheter and also had to walk slowly because of the needle that was in my penis. I was miserable.

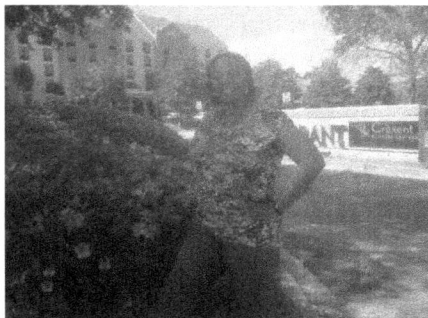

Vikki & I Outside of Hotel

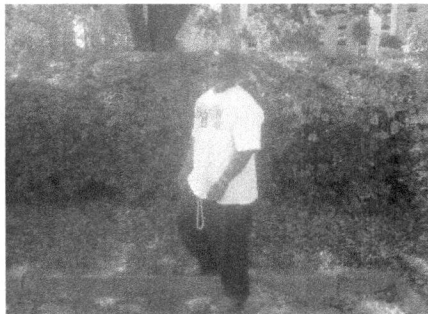

The second day I looked down at my catheter bag, and it was filled with blood. Whenever the bag became full Vikki changed it. I felt helpless. A couple of days later I received a call from my cousin Ann to see how I was doing. I told her I felt about as well to be expected. She asked what hotel I staying, and I told her. She stated, "Well, I just called to see how you were coming along." The next thing I knew, I heard a knock on the door. I became agitated because I thought Vikki had left the room without her hotel key. When I was just about to get up and open the door, Ann walked in laughing. She was with her crew, Angela and Vivian.

Ann and her crew stayed a little while and asked if I wanted anything to eat. I told her that I wanted some ribs and vegetables. Ann went somewhere close to the hotel and brought back plenty of food. After we ate, Ann and her crew went back to Atlanta. The only thing that made my stay out of the hospital bearable was the NBA playoffs that were on television. I knew Vikki was tired because she had to be my sole caregiver. I felt like a child because I had to stand up while she drained my catheter bag. I felt vulnerable because I couldn't move like I wanted to, and if an

144

emergency had happened, I couldn't run or do anything because of the catheter. The next week I returned to the Mayo Clinic to have the catheter removed. I was able to use the restroom on my own. I was very happy. Then my girlfriend and I went back to Orlando where I could finish recovering. To my surprise I was able to do more than I thought that I would be able to do. I didn't experience a lot of incontinence, and when I did, it was off and on for about two weeks. Finally I was able to begin an exercise regimen without using weights. Today is August 18, 2014, and I thank God I'm still cancer free.

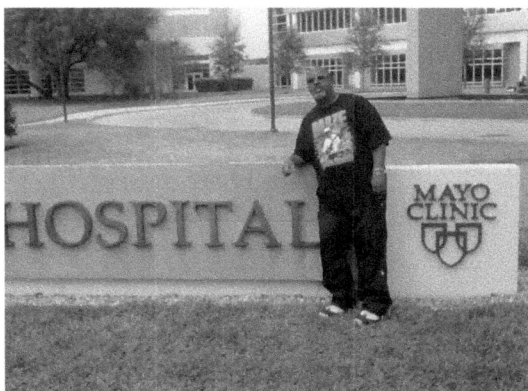

Chillin' at the Mayo Clinic

This Book is Dedicated to
Lieutenant Eric Caldwell, Jr.

You came into my life in 1995. A friendship was created that would forever be embedded in my heart. Your kindness and selfless acts touched my soul. When the government came after me in a hostile way, you encouraged me not to give up; when the government took my money you replenished my account and never asked to be repaid; when I needed a friend to talk to you lent your ear.

When we first met on the job, you let me know that you were in charge at the Federal Correctional Institution Tallahassee. Caldwell you had a work ethic that was second to none. You always worked with high standards of professionalism!

You took your career seriously and I admired you for this. I learned from you, I saw you as a mentor and as a role model for any young man or woman seeking to succeed! Caldwell you were my friend and my big brother. You were big in every way, you were a gentle giant and you left a lasting impression on all who ever met you. It has been stated that a friend loves at all times and you did exactly that. It pains me to talk about you in the past tense.

On November 18, 2015 I received a call from Officer Susian Hawkins about you. She was kind enough to ask me two questions: she asked, if I was sitting down and was anyone at home with me.

She cared enough about me to know that what she was going to tell me was going to crush me and when she dropped the news of your death, my knees buckled. I was heartbroken and refused to believe my best friend in Florida was gone. I said, 'If our other best friend Lieutenant Walkerfountaine didn't call me and inform me of your death, then the news I received from Officer Hawkins couldn't be true.'

Instantly, I went to the telephone and called Walkerfountaine to ask her had she heard the news, when she picked up her phone, she said in a very upbeat voice, "What's up G, how are you doing?"

She went on to say, "G, I just arrived back from Houston, Texas and Caldwell came to the airport and picked me up and he is still angry about the doctors giving him the run around about his health, they have misdiagnosed him for 19 months and he is tired of it. As a matter of fact G, he has obtained a lawyer and today I'm going to assist him with his paperwork."

"Caldwell, after I finished talking to Lieutenant Walkerfountaine I came to realize she didn't have a clue that you had passed away. Caldwell it was your strength in the past that showed me I could function in the face of tragedy." With that said, I had to break the bad news to Walkerfountaine about your death; needless to say she was devastated.

It was Walkerfountaine and your wife, Patricia Ann, who witnessed your health declining while doctors could not figure out what was amiss.

It was more frustrating when the insurance company refused to pay for you to go seek other specialist about your condition. Patricia Ann and Walkerfountaine had to listen to the doctors tell you that nothing was wrong when you knew something on the inside of your body wasn't functioning right.

"Although I haven't come to terms about your death, I do know one thing, God makes no mistakes and as long as I live, I will make sure your death was not in vain."

"Caldwell, we always shared quality time, therefore I have no regrets on 'time' now that you're gone. Some people regret not sharing quality time with loved ones, but not in this case. There wasn't a time when I was in Tallahassee that we didn't see each other. There wasn't a time I didn't enjoy our conversation via the telephone."

I will never forget when you attended my retirement party, you told me, "G, don't go to the city and forget about me," and I told you, "Once I accept you as a friend we would be in communication until the end."

Again, we would never have imagined that we would lose you in such a short span of time, but God knows best. May you rest in peace and from all your labor.

Your Friend,

Lieutenant Garry L. Jones

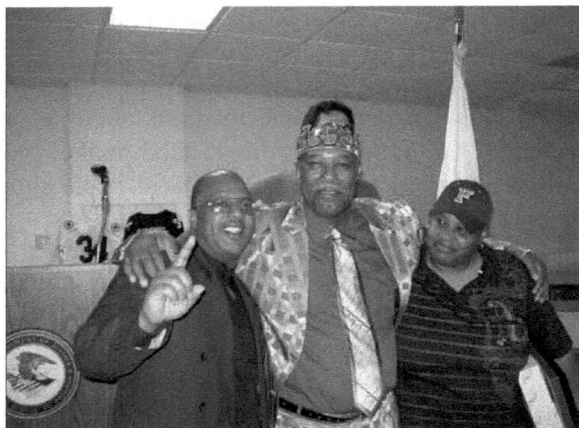

Lt. Jones (me), Lt. Caldwell, and Lt. Walkerfountaine at Lt. Caldwell's Retirement Ceremony from the Federal Bureau of Prisons

www.ingramcontent.com/pod-product-compliance
Lightning Source LLC
Chambersburg PA
CBHW070732220326
41598CB00024BA/3396